PRAISE [illegible]

YOUR LONGEVITY BLUEPRINT

"Whether you are newly diagnosed or a patient who continues to struggle with a long list of confusing symptoms, Your Longevity Blueprint *will be a helpful guide in your journey to reclaim your health and vitality."*

—Terry Wahls, MD. Author of the *Wahls Protocol: A Radical New Way to Treat All Chronic Autoimmune Conditions.*

"Your Longevity Blueprint *is the road map to aging healthier. It bridges the gap between conventional medicine and alternative methodologies. Most importantly, this book understands that to change healthcare we need the patient's involvement.* Your Longevity Blueprint *guides patients to building a healthier body so they can participate in their healthcare and avoid being overmedicated and overdiagnosed."*

—Gary S. Donovitz, MD, FACOG. CEO and Medical Director of BioTE Medical, LLC.

"Dr. Gray skillfully guides you through a comprehensive system to alleviate resistant symptoms and improve your health and quality of life. Following this blueprint will empower you and give you the ability to live a longer and healthier life."

—Dr. Joseph Collins, ND, RN. Author of *Discover Your Menopause Type.*

"Dr. Stephanie Gray's Your Longevity Blueprint *is an extremely well-thought-out, well-researched guide for patients who are looking to take a more functional or personalized approach to their wellness. This book will help them understand each area of their health, and will provide important tools to make positive changes when they have been told everything is 'fine' when it is not."*

—Carrie Jones, ND, MPH. Medical Director of Precision Analytical, Inc.

"One of the greatest challenges in our society today as it relates to understanding and treating chronic health issues is weeding through the mountain of information and deciding what is relevant to the issue at hand in each individual. In her book, Dr. Gray not only does a great job bringing forth the relevant information, but she breaks it down into relatable terms that are easy to understand and apply."

—Thomas Houle, BS. Ortho Molecular Products.

"Dr. Stephanie Gray's wisdom into health has helped so many people, and this book takes the health we all know and breaks it down to fully uncover the root problems in our own individual lives. Your Longevity Blueprint *is a guide to take what is known and find the culprit, helping you to find healing. This book is helpful, honest, and hopeful."*

—Alexa Schirm, Simple Roots Wellness.

YOUR LONGEVITY
BLUEPRINT

BUILDING A HEALTHIER BODY THROUGH
FUNCTIONAL MEDICINE

YOUR LONGEVITY BLUEPRINT

DR. STEPHANIE GRAY

Advantage®

Published by Advantage, Charleston, South Carolina.
Member of Advantage Media Group.

Printed in the United States of America.

10 9 8 7 6 5 4 3 2 1

ISBN: 978-1-59932-859-1
LCCN: 2017959650

Cover design by George Stevens.
Graphics by Melanie Cloth.
Layout design by Megan Elger.

This book is dedicated to all my patients—past, present, and future.
Thank you for letting me be your guide.

DISCLAIMER

The information provided in this book is intended to educate persons on health care and related issues that may affect their daily lives. No information in this book should be considered to be—or used as a substitute for—medical advice, diagnosis, or treatment. To the fullest extent permitted by law, the author, Integrative Health and Hormone Clinic, Inc., and Your Longevity Blueprint disclaims any representations or warranties that any products or health strategies mentioned in this book are safe, appropriate, or effective for the reader. The author advises the reader to always seek the advice of a physician or other qualified health care provider with any questions regarding personal health or medical conditions. In no event shall the author, Integrative Health and Hormone Clinic, Inc., or Your Longevity Blueprint be liable for any direct, indirect, incidental, consequential, special, exemplary, punitive, or any other monetary or other damages arising out of or relating in any way to the information provided in this book.

TABLE OF CONTENTS

ACKNOWLEDGMENTS

First and foremost I must thank my Savior, Jesus Christ. He has instilled in me my passion for health. He has sustained me through all my life's challenges, including my health issues and building our practice.

Secondly, I'd like to thank my husband, Eric Gray. He proposed, I started a clinic at the young age of twenty-eight, and one year later we were married. He eventually resigned from his job to come manage the practice. He has made several sacrifices to honor my passions and my dreams and to support our clinic's goals. He has provided me with unconditional love, even through our most stressful years when I returned to graduate school for a second and third time while working more than full time.

Eric, you are my rock and my biggest cheerleader. You deserve more than I can write in this acknowledgment. You are the most amazing example of God's gifting and plan for my life.

Thank you to my parents who have always lifted me up and believed in me. Thank you for raising us in a healthy home. Dad, thank you for instilling in me an entrepreneurial spirit. Your optimism is contagious. Mom, thank you for consistently reading to me, including the children's book by Dr. Seuss, *Oh, the Places You'll Go,* over and over as a child, teaching me to dream big.

Thank you to my brothers Ricky and Shaun who have always been there to cheer me on, support me, and provide a laugh when needed.

Thank you to my godparents, Dr. Michael Brooks, MD, and his wife, Vicki, for always providing me a spiritual home base (along with my parents) for all my decisions.

Thanks to all the staff we've had at our clinic from the beginning. We love our team and couldn't provide the care we do without you all.

Thank you to the late Richard Noyes, MD, and his wife, Martha, for your generosity in helping provide me a location in our first year of operation.

I'd also like to thank all my mentors from the beginning: Dr. Joseph Collins, ND, RN, the American Academy of Anti-Aging Medicine, Dr. Gary Donovitz, MD, BioTE, Lenchen Raeside, and my colleagues and instructors at the University of Iowa College of Nursing.

Thank you, Dr. Calla Jayne Kleene, DC, for your incredible passion as chiropractor, your loyal friendship, honest feedback, and endless encouragement. It was an honor to have you write the foreword for this book.

Thank you to everyone who has prayed for us and helped our business grow from our humble beginnings and into our future.

ABOUT THE AUTHOR

Dr. Stephanie Gray, DNP, MS, ARNP, ANP-C, GNP-C, ABAAHP, FAARFM, has been a nurse practitioner since 2009. With a doctorate from the University of Iowa and a master's from the University of South Florida's Medical School, Dr. Gray's expertise lies in integrative, anti-aging, and functional medicine. Objectively one of the Midwest's most credentialed female healthcare providers, she was the first nurse practitioner in Iowa certified through the American Academy of Anti-Aging Medicine Board of Anti-Aging Health Practitioners (ABAAHP), and she also completed the Advanced Fellowship in Anti-Aging, Regenerative, and Functional Medicine through the American Academy of Anti-Aging Medicine in 2013. Also in 2013, Dr. Gray became the first BioTE certified provider in the state of Iowa to administer hormone pellets. She continues to stay progressive with the study of natural hormone replacement therapy and nutrigenomics. This training allows her to provide patients with the most comprehensive care. She is also the author of the Higher Learning Technologies' app, FNP (Family Nurse Practitioner) Mastery, available for download on the iTunes App Store. She and her husband, Eric, own the Integrative Health and Hormone Clinic in Cedar Rapids, Iowa.

FOREWORD

I first met Dr. Stephanie Gray in 2009 at a local Professional Women's Network (PWN) lunch-in and chapter meeting. She was the presenting guest speaker, leading a talk about preventative medicine and women's health. I only attended because I read her bio in an email chain promoting the event. I was immediately infatuated with a "medical" provider that indicated she may slant a little into the "all-natural" world that I love as a chiropractor. I had no idea that her presentation would move me in such a way that it would change my own trajectory personally and professionally. I also believe it was one of those "open door" opportunities that God hands us every once in a while. I just didn't know it at the time. Typically I don't stay behind and meet presenters or kiss face after presentations I dig, because I feel the presenter has better things to do, or because I'm really "not that important" anyway. Thank God I did something different the day I heard Dr. Stephanie Gray speak.

In 2009, I had just opened my own chiropractic office in Hiawatha, Iowa. I can't remember exactly how our conversation went after I shook her hand and introduced myself to this amazingly passionate and insanely smart professional. I pretty much smiled and shook my head in agreement at literally everything she was presenting on.

Being fresh out of chiropractic school, a lot of my own professional dogma was geared more toward "anti-medicine," no matter what the scenario. My own ignorance probably had more weight as well, and I don't mean to stereotype all chiropractors, but what Dr. Gray was sharing with the group of women was so foundational in true health, true wellness, and was truly preventative. Her message helped connect the "all-natural" (complementary and alternative) world with the "science is medicine" world. She had the passion for all things natural and the brains for patient-specific data (labs) to support her natural methods.

Not only did her first-born, type A personality have insane sources for all of her claims and data, but she went well above the care of the general audience listening to her present that day.

She would later encourage me to join her at an "anti-aging" conference. I put it off for a few years, because when I jumped on the website I was jaded by the term "anti-aging" medicine. I knee-jerked in offense that anti-aging was more aesthetic. Being twenty-four years old at the time, I was working on appearing older so my patients and my community would take me more seriously. Don't worry, now at thirty-two years old I'm thinking, "Of course I want to look younger. Sign me up!" It took me a while before I became full-on in love with functional medicine, especially as it 100 percent complemented my chiropractic backbone.

I finally succumbed and joined Dr. Gray, and we together completed our fellowship in "anti-aging" and regenerative medicine, graduating together in December 2013. During our coursework and seminars, Dr. Gray had this uncanny ability to ask some of the most intense questions that would often stump experts in the functional medicine field. She is also the type that would have read the books and publications of any of our presenters before each seminar, on top of our countless hours of studying and preparing for our exams and fellowship completion. I don't think she made time for sleep in her intense dedication to constant studying and understanding of health. She is intense, and fierce, and sometimes downright intimidating with her level of dedication. Her deep and palpable quest for knowledge is very apparent. At the sacrifice of her own health, Dr. Gray would stay up late and arrive early to her office to make sure her patient charts had been reviewed with great intensity and with a very particular game plan set into motion for every single patient.

When reading her book, *Your Longevity Blueprint*, I could hear and feel her deep conviction and passion for sharing this information. A ton of sweat, blood, and tears went into the development of this book. *Your Longevity Blueprint* has been a dream come true for Dr. Gray because her passion is so great and this allows her to reach a much greater audience. No matter if you are a patient who's new to functional medicine, a nurse, a chiropractor, a medical student, or even a healthcare provider, we all have much to gain from Dr. Gray's blueprint. God has blessed her with such intensity, desire, and passion, and she is doing this work to honor Him.

Incorporating this book and her suggestions will have a affect your health profoundly. I encourage you to read this book, incorporate her suggestions, and then share this book with five of your most favorite people in your life. Everyone deserves health. #wellnessiswaiting

Calla Jayne Kleene, DC
Founder, Back in Line Family Chiropractic in Hiawatha, Iowa
Cofounder, Well Labs

INTRODUCTION

For a mom, health may mean enjoying her children without pain, headaches, or exhaustive fatigue. For a teenage girl, health may mean not succumbing to birth control for her heavy period cycles and PMS. For a father whose memory and stamina are declining, health may be the ability to keep his job.

We all experience times when our health is in question. Sometimes the answers are smacking us in the face, such as losing weight, exercising, and eating clean. Other times, the answers are far more elusive. This book is meant to shed light on answers that may be eluding you. It's intended to provide you with innovative findings and groundbreaking information that is being used within functional medicine today, an approach that should be leading our health care to a paradigm shift.

For most of my life, I appeared to be the embodiment of "perfect" health. I always ate healthy and exercised, and I did not have chronic diseases or conditions such as diabetes, cardiovascular disease, or cancer. Yet at age thirty, two years after starting a private practice, I started suffering from various symptoms, the most challenging of which was tachycardic (fast heart rate) episodes, which interfered with my ability to do my job and kept me up at night, severely impacting my sleep. I was dizzy, short of breath, exhausted, and desperate. I could no longer operate at the high pace I had started my own practice with. Since I was the only clinician practicing within our clinic, my entire team depended on my ability to treat patients effectively and efficiently.

As a clinician trying to guide others toward healing, few knew of my internal struggle. It wasn't something readily seen, but it was challenging nonetheless. Throughout this book, I'll be sharing bits of my personal story to help you see that I can relate to your struggle.

Conventional medicine had no answers for me other than, "Take this medication to control your heart rate." I knew there had to be a better answer. Taking the medication wouldn't tell me "why" this was happening to me.

I was born and raised in the Midwest and grew up in what I considered to be a very healthy family. We regularly went to the chiropractor, we ate clean, home-cooked meals, we took daily vitamins, and we were almost always engaged in some type of physical activity. It was a rare treat for my brothers and I to eat something containing sugar; I still recall one brother stealing a spoonful of sugar from the kitchen, then hiding behind our couch just to eat that sweet treat. If that isn't a clear indication of how powerful and addictive sugar can be, then I don't know what is. One of my family's favorite stories from my childhood was my first lemonade stand. I couldn't quite understand why no one liked my lemonade until I found out that one of the key ingredients was—what else—sugar. Since I had such limited exposure to sugar, I hadn't added any to my batch. No wonder everyone found it to be a tad sour.

From a young age, I had a thirst for knowledge, an eagerness to understand all that life has to offer, and a desire to achieve. Cheerleading, volleyball, soccer, piano and flute lessons, baton, gymnastics, diving, orchestra, dance, and show choir occupied my childhood and high school years—and that doesn't even include any of my academic pursuits. My inquisitive behavior and desire to succeed carried over into my adult years and became a true strength in my quest for understanding the human condition physically, mentally, and spiritually. Those early years shaped who I am today, not only in relation to my eating and exercise habits, but also to my work ethic, and my desire to help others achieve their health goals.

I felt called to enter the health care field right out of high school, so I entered college with the intention of becoming a radiology technician—but after only one semester I realized that wasn't my purpose. That's when I began considering either nursing or medical school, in the end choosing holistic nursing as my future. I was inspired by its focus on the whole human body, treating the biological, psychological, social, cultural, and spiritual self simply made the most sense. Even then, I knew that healing requires more than just focusing on anatomy. As a social butterfly growing up, I saw how close relationships, or lack thereof, could greatly impact the ability to heal. My upbringing in church and putting God at the center of my life also helped me understand the integral role that spirituality plays in healing.

Holistic nursing theory appreciates and emphasizes that healing must encompass the interconnectedness of the mind, body, and spirit, but must also include emotions, relationships, and environment. This ideology has shaped and remained at the forefront of my private practice today.

My first "revelation" in nursing came while working in a nursing home as a certified nursing assistant (CNA) with patients who had trouble controlling their bladders (incontinence). I was disappointed by the level of care that residents at the nursing home received—for example, they often would lie for hours in urine-soaked clothes or briefs, sometimes even through the night, until one of the few CNAs on staff had time to change them. To be clear, I know how hard the staff in nursing facilities works, and I know it's nearly impossible for CNAs to keep up through the night, because incontinence is so prevalent. In fact, I discovered that incontinence is one of the main reasons people are admitted to long-term care facilities. That led me to believe that if I could somehow improve bladder control, then I could improve the residents' quality of life and quite possibly help reduce admissions to these facilities for some people altogether. I decided to become a certified continence nurse. Soon I discovered that conventional medicine basically approached incontinence with only two options: drugs and surgery. Through my training, however, I learned that incontinence can also be improved with bladder retraining, diet changes, pelvic floor muscle exercises, and even pessary devices for prolapse.

These are nonpharmacological, nonsurgical options that many patients are not being introduced to. Incontinence and pessary fittings may not be the first topic that comes to mind when people think of the "functional" or "integrative" medicine approach, but that was my watershed moment. That's when I first realized that the American health care system was failing a group of people with one of the most basic ailments. In truth, there are few examples of functionality better than a person who regains their independence after a simple pessary fitting has improved their continence. To date, I'm thankful for my continence certification and for learning how to fit patients with pessaries. It is still a service that I offer at my clinic, and it has truly changed patients' lives.

Once I found nonsurgical, nonpharmacological ways to treat incontinence, I knew there had to also exist ways to treat other ailments or disease states from this perspective. That's when I decided that if I was going to work in health care, I needed to work in a way that held true to my belief systems, both from my upbringing, and from what I learned in nursing training. I absolutely love being a nurse, and there is no better feeling than caring for others. I also love facing and overcoming new challenges, and my ultimate goal at the time was to become a nurse practitioner (NP).

So, upon completion of my bachelor of science in nursing, I went on to graduate school to become a nurse practitioner. I was one of the youngest nurses in the program, but that only fueled my desire, because it meant that I would spend nearly my entire adult life in service to others.

Since my parents were so open to natural methods of achieving and maintaining health and preventing disease, I knew I wanted to eventually incorporate a more natural approach into my own practice. I knew I needed to obtain additional, *different* training, but I wasn't quite sure where to turn next. In my final clinical semester of school, I shadowed a nurse practitioner who owned a private practice. One day, a nutraceutical representative stopped in to explain a seven-day liver detox. It was a new concept to me, but I was easily convinced that it was something worth trying. The week of the detox, I felt amazingly better, because I eliminated the topmost allergenic foods—gluten, eggs, soy, corn, peanuts, fish, and dairy—and I ate only organic. My brain fog lifted, I lost seven pounds, and I gained more energy. I know now that much of what I experienced in the detox was the result of removing gluten from my diet, because, as I learned, I have a sensitivity to it.

The detox was a small but important step in my growth as an advanced registered nurse practitioner (ARNP). It helped me to see that a different way of practicing medicine existed, but I still didn't quite know how to tap into that knowledge base.

When I entered practice as an NP, one of my first patients gave me a *Life Extension* magazine that included an advertisement for an American Academy of Anti-Aging Medicine (A4M) conference only a few months away. I booked my flight, and the rest is history. After that first conference, I attended one or two more of them per year, along with other annual events and bioidentical hormone seminars. Over time, I completed the Health Care Diplomat program and the Advanced Fellowship in Anti-Aging, Regenerative, and Functional Medicine (now available through the Metabolic Medical Institute [MMI] as an Advanced Fellowship in Metabolic, Nutritional and Functional Medicine). At the time, I was one of only two advanced fellows in my state. I also completed a master's in metabolic nutritional medicine through the University of South Florida Medical School, which partners with MMI. That training taught me how to truly help patients improve their health.

The primary way I offer this is through the Integrative Health and Hormone Clinic in Cedar Rapids, Iowa, that I own with my husband, Eric. Through my experience as a practitioner and my personal health struggles, I've developed a unique way of viewing how the human body is structured. It's been quite a journey growing our practice while regaining and maintaining my health.

Like me, many patients, dissatisfied with a lack of answers from conventional medicine, seek help through homeopathic, integrative, restorative, chiropractic, antiaging, alternative, or functional medicine. I chose to pursue integrative and functional medicine simply because it was the first approach outside my conventional training that I was exposed to. The bottom line is that it's not as much about the terminology as it is about the core principles the practitioner follows.

Patrick Flynn, DC, owner of the Wellness Way Clinic, has a unique illustration for current differences in health care, which he describes as the fireman-versus-carpenter approach. In his comparison, conventional medicine is the fire department—it is needed to "put out fires" that erupt in a person's health. The fire department extinguishes fires using only an axe and a hose— these are the drugs and surgery used in conventional medicine. Although conventional medicine is an important part of health care, patients typically aren't taught how to find and fix the "faulty circuitry" that started the fire in the first place. The carpenter approach, on the other hand, helps patients repair and rebuild the body—similar to how a carpenter rebuilds a home after a fire. Getting the body and all of its organ systems back to optimal functionality is the true definition of health, and it's the basis of functional medicine. Functional medicine also looks at the interactions of nutrition, genetics, hormones, toxins, and infections (many of which will be discussed in this book).

Functional medicine asks how and why illness occurs and restores health by addressing the root cause of the disease (IFM.org). Integrative medicine integrates or combines conventional medicine with complementary and alternative methods. Conventional medicine is needed at times, but often patients need more. I needed more. I practice both integrative and functional medicine, because I integrate conventional medicine with natural methods, working to address the root cause of the disease. I wrote this book to help patients better understand functional medicine, but also to help other providers struggling with decisions about what to do for their patients.

Patients commonly tell me their "regular" doctor or internist "says it's all in my head." Many clinicians want to help their patients, but they simply do not know all the options that are available. They may have taken one weekend course on gut health and on that basis think they've got a handle on the gastrointestinal system. But that's only one aspect of restoring health.

As conventional medicine continues to fail patients, many of them are becoming their own advocates. Conventional medicine failed me, too, when my own health became an issue. I, too, have struggled with symptoms that conventional medicine couldn't find a root cause for. That's how I came to realize that it's my calling to share what I know can be a better road to healing.

That's when I decided a blueprint was needed, and my personal struggles have helped me create it. Patients and providers need a "Longevity Blueprint." Regardless of the symptoms—headaches, irritable bowel syndrome, psoriasis, tachycardia, or fatigue—this blueprint will help.

There have been many books written on how important adopting a stress-free lifestyle truly is. You can easily find books written on dieting, yoga, stretching, meditation, optimizing your sleep, and the importance of proper exercise. I have benefited from many of these that offer help in reducing stress. Since I believe all of these subjects are extremely important, I talk to my patients about them daily, and what I've found is that many individuals are already doing many of these activities and are still, well, sick.

If you're reading this book, I'm assuming you're already trying some of these mentioned strong health habits. You're sleeping well, incorporating stress-reduction techniques, and exercising, and you want to build a healthier body. This book is for individuals who are struggling to find answers to their health issues, and for those who want to take their health to the next level. It's for people who want the best quality of life—*longevity*!

The following chapters contain a blueprint created to help build your personal longevity. Each chapter discusses how your organs and the systems of the body work together to build your longevity. It's a bit like building a home—you need a blueprint to ensure the final outcome is a place you can live for a long time. With your body, you need a blueprint to ensure that every aspect is addressed in order to have a long and healthy life.

Within each of the following chapters, I share the most progressive available functional medicine testing options, as well as our Longevity Blueprint (LB) nutraceutical products, which we use at my clinic. Our brand is evidence based. We've created formulations that work. We have the highest standards for our raw materials, and we use only the most therapeutic potencies. Just as human fingerprints are detailed, unique markers of human identity, so are your test results. These will help your health care provider personalize a plan to build your health.

Since your gut is the foundation to your overall health, the first chapter is very comprehensive. My goal in this book is that you as the reader, patient, or provider will be able to address one particular function in your house (organ system in your body)—especially if it's a system that you are struggling to understand or find solutions for. I want you to be able to address each system in your body (each function in your house) to achieve optimal longevity.

I will also offer resources for aging well. The best is yet to come, whether you are thirty-three or ninety-three.

Everyone is at a different point in their health journey. Regardless of where you are, this book has a wealth of information to help you get better or stay better.

Wellness is Waiting™! Let's get started!

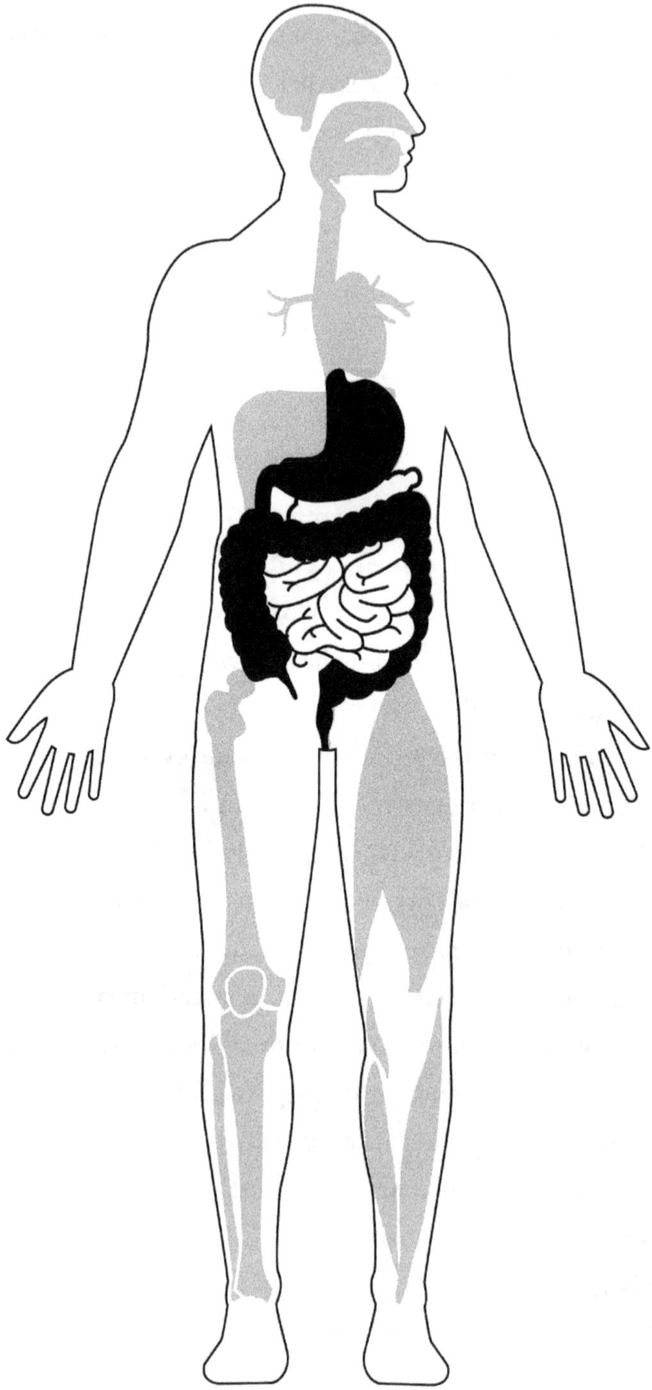

CHAPTER 1

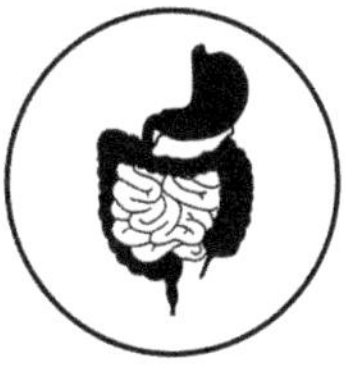

YOUR FOUNDATION: RESTORING GUT HEALTH

Health is "a state of optimal physical, mental, and social well-being, and not merely the absence of disease or infirmities."

—World Health Organization

Jennifer had daily chronic migraines. She missed much of high school because of them, and now was struggling through college, often spending her time heavily medicated and sleeping in her darkened bedroom instead of going to class. She had seen a neurologist for years and had tried numerous migraine medications.

Her bowels had always been normal, so she had never been referred to a gastrointestinal specialist. Neither her primary care provider nor her neurologist ever asked her what she ate on a daily basis.

Jennifer was also a good friend of mine. I witnessed how much of life she missed due to her pain. It wasn't until she finally allowed me to test her for food sensitivities and celiac disease that her life changed.

YOUR GUT, THE FOUNDATION OF YOUR HEALTH

I'm not a home builder, I'm a clinician, but I figure that most people know that the foundation of a house is extremely important. Think about it: the foundation has to support the weight of the entire house. If the house is built on a weak or improperly built foundation, the house can eventually crumble. Have you ever seen the kind of devastation that results from a poorly constructed foundation? It's a costly repair—far more costly than building the foundation right from the start.

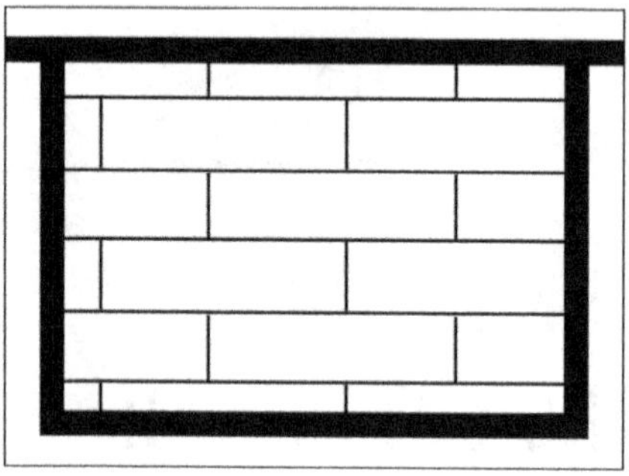

The same is true for the human body—it must have a healthy foundation on which to build good health. The foundation of your body's health is your gut, due in part to the fact that 70 to 80 percent of your immune system lives in your gastrointestinal wall.

In her book *Gut and Psychology Syndrome*, Natasha Campbell-McBride, MD, states that the "gut wall can be described as the right hand of the immune system" (Campbell-McBride 2010, 31). That is one reason why, for instance, having a vaginal delivery and breastfeeding is so important—which we'll discuss in more detail soon. It's important to build a good gastrointestinal microbiome and strong immune system, or foundation, from the beginning stages of life. Our microbiome is defined by *Merriam-Webster's Dictionary* as the collection and community of symbiotic, commensal, and pathogenic bacteria, as well as other microorganisms (such as fungi, and viruses) that inhabit your human body. It's your mini ecosystem.

The establishment of good bacteria must take place within the first three weeks of life or the child can be left with a weak immune system. Beneficial gut bacteria provide protective "walls," without which the body is more susceptible to gastrointestinal infections. Campbell-McBride likens "a well-functioning gut with healthy gut flora" to the roots of a tree—without healthy roots, a tree cannot thrive. The same goes for the body; the "rest of the body cannot thrive without a well-functioning digestive system." The bacteria in the gut—known as the gut flora—is the "soil" that gives the tree, or the body, its "habitat, protection, support, and nourishment" (Campbell-McBride 2010, 25).

In addition to housing our good bacteria, our gut is also important because it helps with our digestion. When proteins are not properly digested, they can appear like the opiates morphine and heroine. The protein gluten—found in wheat, barley, rye, and oats, as well as in the protein casein in milk—can cause that "high" effect. When a person is sensitive to gluten, reducing its consumption can leave them feeling withdrawal symptoms similar to those that occur when withdrawing from opiates.

In *Grain Brain*, author David Perlmutter, MD, more specifically explains that gluten acts as an adhesive material. That's why it is often used in the baking process, as it holds the dough together and allows it to stretch. Foods containing gluten can be more difficult to digest. As Perlmutter explains, gluten's "sticky attribute" can interfere with the absorption of nutrients, as the "pasty residue can alert your immune system to leap into action, eventually resulting in an assault on the lining of the small intestine" (Perlmutter with Loberg 2013, 51).

In the *Immune Recovery Diet*, author Susan Blum, MD, discusses suggestions for patients with autoimmune disease, starting with cleaning up the gut. Blum discusses how foods contain carbs, fats, and proteins. Proteins are made up of amino acids. The body's incredible immune system can recognize different patterns of amino acids, attacking some to rid the body of them while leaving others alone.

Even viruses, yeast, and bacteria have their own amino acid codes. Blum states: "The amino acid sequences are the foundation for how the immune system reads name tags in both foreign and your own cells ... because foods have amino acids they can cause the alarm if your immune cells don't recognize them" (Blum 2013, 44). Through a process known as "molecular mimicry," gluten can resemble other tissue structures in your body. Molecular mimicry is defined as "sequence similarities between foreign and self-peptides that are sufficient to result in the cross-activation of autoreactive T or B cells by pathogen-derived peptides," essentially meaning this is when your body mistakes your own tissue for a foreigner (Blum 2013). So while your body is on alert to attack the gluten, it may also attack other vital organs, such as your thyroid. When the thyroid is inflamed and leaks out thyroid peroxidase enzymes (which look like gluten), a body on alert for gluten may also attack those thyroid enzymes. That creates thyroid peroxidase antibodies, which leads to autoimmune thyroid disease. However, this process doesn't only create autoimmune conditions in the thyroid, it can create other autoimmune conditions, such as multiple sclerosis, rheumatoid arthritis, and others.

In *Wheat Belly*, William Davis, MD, discusses how removing wheat from your diet can help you lose weight, get rid of "man boobs," and reduce insulin resistance. In essence, Davis makes the case for why cleaning up your gut can impact the health of your entire body.

WHAT IS LEAKY GUT?

Many clients have read about the dangers of "leaky gut," or "gastrointestinal (GI) permeability." They come to me wanting to fix/

heal the condition—they want to strengthen their gastrointestinal foundation. So, what is leaky gut?

Think of your gut lining as a strong security system. The enterocyte cells that line the gut should be positioned tightly side by side. It's a little like bricks and mortar in a wall. That lining should permit the absorption of certain nutrients and keep harmful agents out. However, if the layer of cells becomes patchy and gaps begin to develop between cells, harmful substances can leak through the security system.

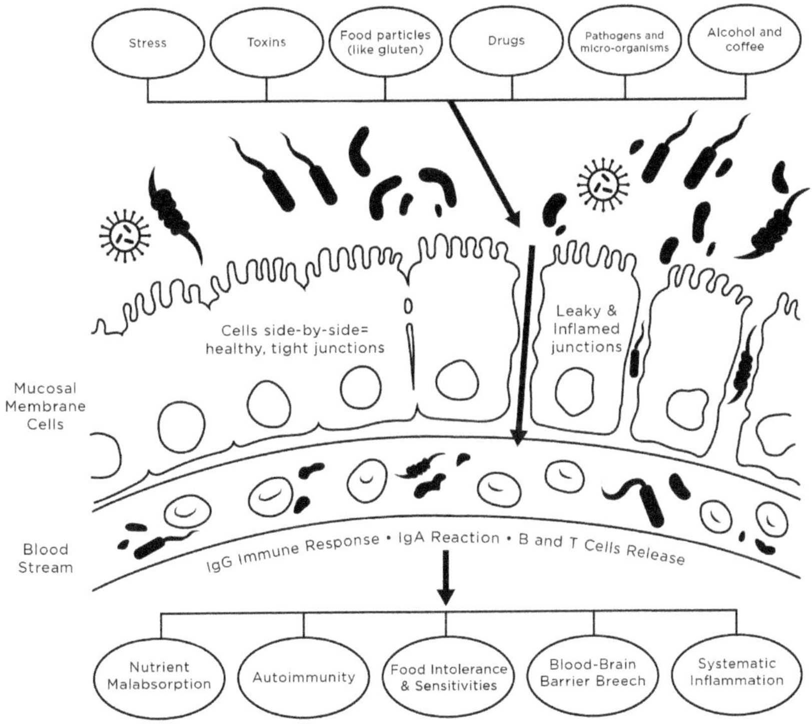

Leaky Gut

How does damage to the wall happen? Damage to the gut lining can occur through various stressors, not just psychologic stress, but also medications like antibiotics, which can destroy good gut bacteria—

not to mention drinking alcohol and coffee, eating processed and genetically modified foods, and eating foods that cause inflammation (which vary from person to person). Even exposure to germs in your daily environment and incurring stress can damage the gut lining. Then what once looked like brick and mortar now just looks like bricks without mortar. Gaps in the wall develop, allowing proteins that are not supposed to make it through the wall to enter into the blood stream. When that happens, the immune system is triggered to attack them. Even worse, it starts attacking what may have once been a good food for you. The immune system marks those food proteins as bad, and creates antibodies to protect you against them.

This can lead to malnourishment, nutritional deficiencies, and even hormonal imbalances, since hormone pathways require these nutrients. And, since your body needs nutrients for the immune cells to function appropriately, it can lead to immune issues. These nutrients are also required for your body to produce energy. In addition, once you have leaky gut, you develop a greater likelihood for food sensitivities. For instance, gluten may have been the biggest trigger for you, but, now that you have leaky gut, the almonds you eat every day are now leaking through the gut barrier into the bloodstream, at which point your body creates antibodies to almonds. Those antibodies will then show up on your food sensitivity testing, even though they weren't the main problem in the first place. The biggest danger is the inflammatory cascade that can occur and cause various symptoms, which are different for each person.

In Jennifer's case, her migraines were caused by inflammation from gluten. In other patients' cases, their skin issues, acne, psoriasis, or even eczema could be a result of inflammation.

HOW DO YOU HEAL LEAKY GUT?

The way to start healing the gut is by eliminating triggering foods, treating infections, and helping to facilitate better digestion and absorption of nutrients. Taking gut-healing nutrients can also help.

The Institute for Functional Medicine teaches clinicians the 5-R Protocol for gut healing:

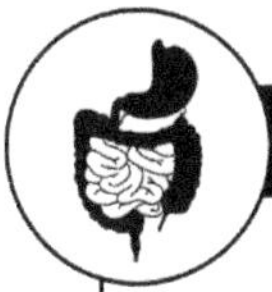

HOW DO YOU HEAL "LEAKY GUT"?

1. REMOVE
(Food sensitivities and gut infections)
2. REPLACE
(Enzymes, HCL, bile)
3. REESTABLISH OR REINOCULATE
(Probiotics and prebiotics)
4. REPAIR
(Glutamine, zinc, omega-3s, and turmeric)
5. REBALANCE
(Manage stress, sleep, and exercise)

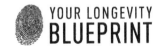

DR. STEPHANIE GRAY YOUR LONGEVITY BLUEPRINT

In the **Remove** phase, the patient removes the common allergy-producing foods, including grains containing gluten and dairy products. In my practice, they also need to remove the foods they react to, identified through testing. Additionally, if the patient is suffering from chronic infections of the sinus, oral cavity, or intestinal tract, these also need to be treated.

During the **Replace** phase, the patient is evaluated for their sufficiency of digestive enzymes and proper stomach acid—again, through testing, as well as through symptom review (such as bloating, gas, and reflux). If these are identified as being a problem, digestive aids such as digestive enzymes, hydrochloric acid, or bile may be recommended with meals.

During the **Reestablish or Reinoculate** phase to improve intestinal immune function and thereby improve whole body function, the patient is typically recommended a therapeutic dose of a combination of probiotics. Additionally, these may be taken with a prebiotic supplement such as inulin, fructooligosaccharides, or arabinogalactans. The patient's actual needs can be evaluated through testing. The reinoculate phase is usually started over a two-week period, during which doses are slowly increased to allow the intestinal tract to adjust. This method can help keep the patient from suffering from excessive intestinal gas formation and discomfort.

During the **Repair** phase, the patient adds nutrient supplements to promote proper repair of the intestinal lining. These typically include the amino acid L-glutamine (6–10 grams per day), zinc citrate (10 mg per day), and omega-3s (1–3 grams per day). Supplements can also involve taking natural anti-inflammatories like turmeric.

During the **Rebalance** phase, additional lifestyle choices are addressed. Sleep, exercise, and stress can all affect the gastrointestinal tract. Taking the time to exercise, considering yoga and meditation for stress reduction, and optimizing sleep are important here.

Think of these five R steps as the footings for your healthy home foundation. This regimen is typically applied for a minimum of twelve weeks. According to the Institute for Functional Medicine (IFM), this regimen "has resulted in tens of thousands of positive outcomes in patients who suffer from many health problems that have resulted from alterations of immune system function and increased inflammation" (www.functionalmedicine.org). If you are a provider and this is new to you, I highly recommend you join the IFM and learn this protocol.

So how is the 5-R Protocol applied? Let's start by looking more specifically at phase 1: Remove. This phase involves (A) removing triggering foods, and (B) removing infections.

PHASE 1A: REMOVE TRIGGERING FOODS

The two main triggers or irritants in the gut are (1) food allergies and sensitivities, and (2) gastrointestinal infections that stress the immune system and cause inflammation. I've had several patients spend hundreds of dollars on gut-healing bone broths or collagen proteins online (which are great products), but have never invested in seeing a functional medicine provider, and thus they have never been able to identify and remove their triggers. Until the triggers are removed, gut healing won't occur.

Foods truly can make a person feel ill. I've had patients who were waking up daily with symptoms such as nausea that were entirely resolved simply by changing their diet. Many individuals assume that diarrhea or constipation are the only symptoms of food sensitivities, while I've had many patients with food sensitivities that have *no* gastrointestinal issues. They, however, have other, atypical symptoms instead.

What happens on your skin may be a reflection of what is happening in your gut. For instance, I have found that inflammatory conditions like eczema and psoriasis are primarily triggered by food sensitivities or infections. I've have patients with acne-like lesions on their head or even hives on their skin who have resolved their symptoms through a change in their diet. Applying a steroid cream or using an antihistamine may help, but that strategy is not getting to the root cause. Additionally, chronic fatigue, joint pains, fibromyalgia, and even chronic respiratory issues like chronic mucous, congestion, and sinusitis can be caused by food sensitivities (Lord and Bralley 2008). What about chronic ear infections in kids? Could this be a dairy sensitivity? Research has shown that it could (Juntti et al. 1999).

How do you know if you have food sensitivities? You can try an elimination diet and then monitor how you feel as you reintroduce each food. Alternately, you can test. A true elimination diet removes corn, dairy, eggs, gluten, white sugar, shellfish, soy, beef, pork, processed meats, coffee, tea, and chocolate. The aim of an elimination diet is to reduce inflammation, identify food triggers, repair leaky gut, and reduce your incoming toxic burden. These foods are avoided for months, and then reintroduced one at a time. The IFM has a free Comprehensive Elimination Diet Guide available for download to its members.

I commonly see patients who have already tried the elimination diet, and who still can't quite narrow down what foods are the most problematic for them. If the patient feels gassy, bloated, and has diarrhea after eating pizza, it is difficult to determine whether the problem is the cheese, the gluten, the yeast, the eggs, the garlic in the crust, the tomato sauce, or other toppings. Some patients have told me their allergist has said they have no allergies, but they continue to struggle and know that certain foods cause certain symptoms for them. For instance, I commonly see patients produce a large amount of mucus after having consumed meals containing dairy, such as yogurt, milk, cottage cheese, or ice cream. Even though the patient did not have a full-blown immunoglobulin E (IgE) allergy to dairy, clearly dairy is causing symptoms. IgE, which we'll discuss in more detail soon, among other reactions, is the most widely recognized food reaction, one that is so severe that it can cause anaphylactic shock and even death. It is often classified as a Type 1 allergic reaction. By exploring other avenues of testing for different immune reactions to foods, positives are often discovered. In my functional medicine practice, I typically use either immunoglobulin G (IgG), or immunoglobulin A (IgA) blood antibody tests to find these reactions.

This testing is often not covered by insurance, since it is still considered "medically unnecessary and experimental" compared to IgE allergy testing. However, most large, functional medicine labs have these food panels available at a reasonable price. And I have found great clinical utility using all of these tests—IgG, IgA, and IgE.

There is no perfect test, but the major difference between an immediate IgE and an IgG or IgA reaction is the complicating factor that IgG and IgA reactions can be delayed by hours to even a week (Lord and Bralley 2008). Also, the IgG and IgA tests are not the painful skin-prick tests that many individuals are familiar with, as would be used in an allergist office. IgG and IgA tests are typically done after gathering blood via the venipuncture or finger-stick process. Many foods can be tested at once. The foods that are commonly tested include:

- egg white and yolk
- milk and cheese
- soy
- gluten grains such as wheat, barley, rye, and oats
- corn
- rice
- shellfish

- various proteins such as beef, chicken, lamb, and pork
- many fruits and vegetables
- coffee
- baker's and brewer's yeast
- sugarcane

Expanded panels can be ordered if the patient is on a specific diet, such as vegetarian. Patients do not have to fast for the test, since it is looking an immune response in the blood. However, if the patient is currently on steroids or other immunosuppressants, those should be taken into consideration, since the medication could suppress the immune response. Results could show as potentially false negatives, or as reactions to a lesser degree than they may have shown had the patient not been on these medications.

Since IgG reactions can take days to manifest, it is also very difficult for individuals to determine what foods are the problem. When I say "reactions," I am referring to any negative symptoms following consumption of foods. A reaction that takes days to occur is known as a chronic delayed hypersensitivity reaction. That is why testing is so valuable. For instance, if an individual eats a banana on Monday but doesn't have a headache until Wednesday, bananas may have been ruled out as a culprit when they actually could have been the trigger.

Like Jennifer at the beginning of the chapter, my youngest brother struggled with migraines for many years. I finally tested him for food sensitivities, and identified eggs and dairy as his two major triggers. Since he removed those from his diet, he has not suffered from a migraine unless he is exposed to eggs or dairy accidentally. However, since he does not have a healthy gastrointestinal foundation, my goal is to help him rebuild it, and then he may be able to successfully reintroduce those foods.

Testing can reveal surprising reactions. Eating organic is certainly better, but some individuals can still have reactions to organic food—I've seen people react to almonds, broccoli, oranges, and even coffee.

Also, if a patient knows that they react to a certain food, we may try having them avoid all the foods in that particular food family. Patients can also gauge what foods they may react to based on other allergies they have. They may have a cross-sensitivity or cross-reaction from other animal proteins, mites, molds, latex, and medicines, not just foods.

For instance, if someone has a latex allergy, I would also recommend they avoid foods in the latex family, because the body may cross-react to a similar protein found in both latex and these latex family foods. These foods include but are not limited to avocado, banana, chestnut, potato, tomato, kiwi, pineapple, and papaya. Individuals who have peanut or soybean allergies should recognize these foods are in the legume family, which includes beans and lentils.

Another example of a potential cross-sensitivity is found with pollen. If pollen causes problems like itchy throat and watery eyes, those reactions may also happen after eating an apple or celery. Why? The proteins found in some fruits are similar to those found in pollen. If the immune system is already on alert for those proteins, it will attack. This is called oral allergy syndrome (OAS).

Many companies that offer food testing also offer a food family or cross-sensitivity guide. In our clinic, we provide this to our patients when our health coach reviews their food sensitivities with them in a nutritional consultation.

FOOD SENSITIVITY SYMPTOMS

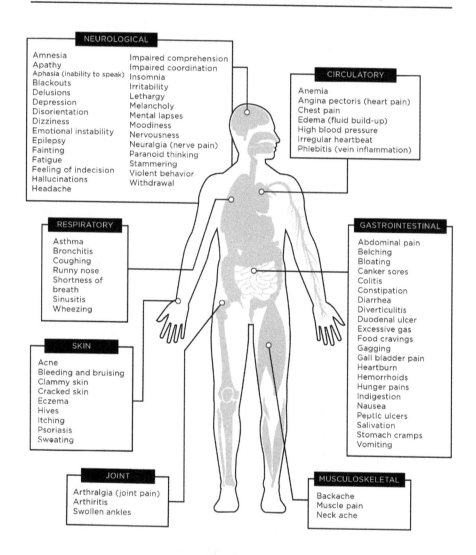

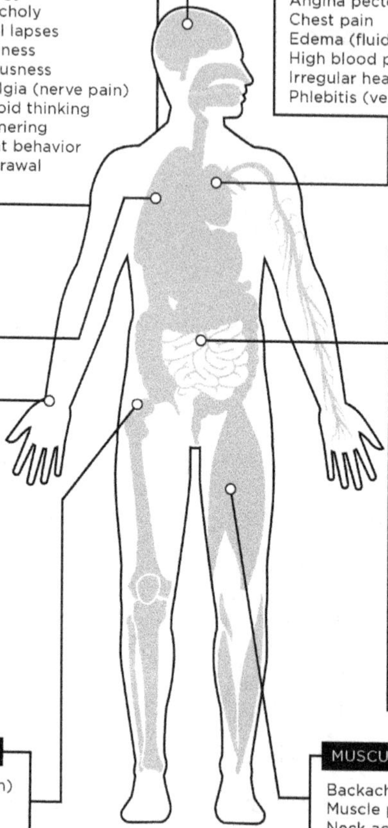

NEUROLOGICAL

- Amnesia
- Apathy
- Aphasia (inability to speak)
- Blackouts
- Delusions
- Depression
- Disorientation
- Dizziness
- Emotional instability
- Epilepsy
- Fainting
- Fatigue
- Feeling of indecision
- Hallucinations
- Headache
- Impaired comprehension
- Impaired coordination
- Insomnia
- Irritability
- Lethargy
- Melancholy
- Mental lapses
- Moodiness
- Nervousness
- Neuralgia (nerve pain)
- Paranoid thinking
- Stammering
- Violent behavior
- Withdrawal

CIRCULATORY

- Anemia
- Angina pectoris (heart pain)
- Chest pain
- Edema (fluid build-up)
- High blood pressure
- Irregular heartbeat
- Phlebitis (vein inflammation)

RESPIRATORY

- Asthma
- Bronchitis
- Coughing
- Runny nose
- Shortness of breath
- Sinusitis
- Wheezing

GASTROINTESTINAL

- Abdominal pain
- Belching
- Bloating
- Canker sores
- Colitis
- Constipation
- Diarrhea
- Diverticulitis
- Duodenal ulcer
- Excessive gas
- Food cravings
- Gagging
- Gall bladder pain
- Heartburn
- Hemorrhoids
- Hunger pains
- Indigestion
- Nausea
- Peptic ulcers
- Salivation
- Stomach cramps
- Vomiting

SKIN

- Acne
- Bleeding and bruising
- Clammy skin
- Cracked skin
- Eczema
- Hives
- Itching
- Psoriasis
- Sweating

JOINT

- Arthralgia (joint pain)
- Arthiritis
- Swollen ankles

MUSCULOSKELETAL

- Backache
- Muscle pain
- Neck ache

OTHER SYMPTOMS

- Bed-wetting
- Cataracts
- Conjunctivitis (swelling of eyelids)
- Diabetes
- Dysmenorrhea (menstrual pain)
- Earaches, ear inflammation, ear discharge
- Failure to thrive in infants
- Fever
- Hoarseness
- Impotence
- Lower blood sugar
- Obesity
- Sneezing spells
- Swelling around eyes
- Tinnitus (ears ringing)

Celiac Disease

Since gluten is a common food trigger, I want to spend some time on this topic. Mayo Clinic defines celiac disease, also known as gluten-sensitive enteropathy, sprue, or coeliac, as, "an immune reaction to eating gluten, a protein found in wheat, barley, and rye" (Mayo Clinic 2017). When a person has celiac disease, eating gluten will trigger an immune response in their small intestine. Over time, as Mayo Clinic states, "this reaction damages your small intestine's lining and prevents absorption of some nutrients (malabsorption). The intestinal damage often causes diarrhea, fatigue, weight loss, bloating, and anemia, and can lead to serious complications" (Mayo Clinic 2017). Children suffering from celiac disease often suffer the same symptoms as adults, but it can also affect their growth and development because of the malabsorption issue. To date, the only way to deal with celiac disease is to follow a strict gluten-free diet, which, "can help manage symptoms and promote intestinal healing" (Mayo Clinic 2017).

Not every patient with celiac disease has diarrhea or constipation. I have had several patients with atypical symptoms of celiac disease. In fact, even infertility can be a symptom of celiac disease. In addition to migraines, Jennifer, my friend mentioned earlier, suffered from endometriosis and infertility in addition to celiac disease. Since she never complained of gastrointestinal symptoms, no provider ever explored foods as a contributing variable and root cause of her illnesses. I tested her for celiac, and her results were some of the strongest I had seen. She was referred for a biopsy, and sure enough, she had severe celiac disease. She has been on a gluten-free diet for years now, so thankfully her migraines are entirely gone, dramatically improving her quality of life. But she has had two laparoscopies for endometriosis, and still has not been able to achieve pregnancy. Yet, I am hopeful that one day she will be able to conceive as she continues to heal her body and reduce overall inflammation.

Her situation, sadly, is typical of many. Additionally, one food sensitivity leading to intestinal permeability leaves a person at a greater likelihood of having more food sensitivities. Jennifer, for instance, also has dairy and egg sensitivities. To help expedite the healing process of her gut, she removed both eggs and dairy short term. But she will remain gluten-free for life.

I never suffered from obvious symptoms of celiac disease. I only tested for it after I had grown desperate because of my tachycardia. My celiac testing was weakly positive, but a positive nonetheless. Although my biopsy was negative, I strongly believe I was clearly on the way to having damage had I continued to ingest gluten. Taking gluten out of my life was my first step toward eradicating my heart palpitation episodes. Diet changes were not once mentioned by my cardiologist.

What are the commonly accepted tests for celiac disease? The gold standard is now tissue transglutaminase antibody IgG in blood and a positive biopsy. I run a full celiac panel on my patients. However, if the blood work is positive—even if the biopsy is negative—the treatment is the same—a gluten-free diet!

Genetic testing is also available. The HLA DQ2 and HLA DQ8 are markers for gluten sensitivity and celiac disease. I actually knew years before my celiac testing was positive that I had these genes. I had already reduced 80 percent of the gluten in my diet, but it was not until I cut it out entirely that my health started to improve.

Of course, if anyone in a family has been diagnosed with celiac disease, then all family members should be tested. I advised one of my first severely celiac female patients to have her two young daughters tested, and sure enough both were positive, and not just genetically—their celiac panel was also positive. One of her daughters wasn't very symptomatic at the time, but unfortunately the other was. That knowledge was truly empowering to the family, however. By changing their diet, they were likely able to avoid many complications and symptoms down the road.

As Davis discusses in *Wheat Belly*, wheat has become a popular part of our diet, especially with processed frozen foods made for our convenience. However, wheat is now very often genetically altered, and those minute differences are likely what is triggering our immune systems. He gives old strands of wheat much credit, but he blames genetic modification for an odd assortment of symptoms—again, likely due to the immune reaction. The body is trying to figure out what the foreign proteins are, and, as a result, keeps the immune system on high alert. For that reason, he recommends a "radical wheat-ectomy," or a total removal of wheat from the diet.

Do you think you are immune? The estimated prevalence of celiac disease is now around 1 percent worldwide. That means 1 in 100 to 133 people have this full-blown autoimmune disease (Gujral, Freeman, and Thomson 2012). The estimated prevalence of people with food allergies (other than gluten) is also on the rise. Many believe that this is at least in part due to genetically modified foods. The estimated prevalence of food allergies is 8 percent in children, and 4 percent in adults (foodallergy.org). I believe this is a low estimate. I'd generally estimate that 90 percent of the patients I have tested (due to symptoms) have sensitivities improved by removing their reactive foods from their diet. Also, 3 percent of the US population is estimated to have autoimmunity; it seems likely that far more have unknown leaky guts, and therefore an even higher prevalence of food sensitivities (IANR 2017). Autoimmune diseases are among the leading causes of death among young and middle-aged women in the United States (Walsh and Rau 2000). Looking into food sensitivities and improving intestinal permeability is one of the best steps toward improving these patients' lives. As Terry Wahls, MD, says, "With autoimmunity...the wires get crossed and, for some unknown reason, the immune cells mistake proteins that are genuinely 'self' as foreign, and more specifically as 'not self and dangerous'" (Wahls 2014).

Not everyone who has a gluten sensitivity has celiac disease. I believe I started with a gluten sensitivity that grew and was on the way to becoming celiac disease, which hopefully I have halted.

At times, it can be difficult to detect food sensitivities. Sometimes, a person's immune system is so besieged that it becomes stressed and worn out. Through the years, I have had patients with obvious symptoms of celiac disease who tested negative to the basic celiac testing their provider ordered. If a total IgA test is not run with a celiac panel, the test result can be a false negative. That means if the patient doesn't have strong immunity—not enough total IgA—they cannot mount a response to gluten, and the tissue transglutaminase IgA may not show on the blood testing. I often test for **total IgA** and **secretory IgA** in my patients, which helps reflect how strong the immune system is specifically along mucous membranes.

Total IgA is a first line of defense for infections along mucosal surfaces. According to Quest Diagnostics, IgA deficiency is more common than may be thought, at 1/400 to 1/700 individuals (Quest Diagnostics 2017). For that reason, if the patient experiences symptoms when consuming certain foods—results of testing aside—they should avoid those foods. If a patient does have a total IgA test run and they are low, their celiac testing will not be conclusive, and will possibly produce a false negative as well. Additionally, **secretory IgA** can also be tested.

When the healthy gastrointestinal flora (good bacteria) is compromised, the ability to produce IgA is reduced. Thus, total IgA is an indirect marker of how well the immune system is doing. You should have ample total IgA and secretory IgA. With that being said, if you don't have enough total IgA your food testing could also produce a false negative. However, this deficiency is much rarer.

Let us go momentarily back to wheat. In discussing the complications of wheat consumption, I must not neglect discussing how addicting this substance can be. As Davis says, the reason that wheat is so addicting is because, upon digestion, it is broken down into polypeptides, which can cross the blood-brain barrier and bind to opiate receptors.

In terms of addiction, wheat is actually very similar to sugar. An article in *Forbes* in 2013 titled, "Research Shows Cocaine And Heroin Are Less Addictive Than Oreos," shows that in clinical trials sugar has even been proven to be as addictive as cocaine (Sullum 2013). I believe it! So it stands to reason that removing wheat from your diet can result in symptoms of withdrawal. These symptoms can include fatigue, mental fog, headaches, nausea, vomiting, and irritability—symptoms that can make it difficult to get through a workday. Davis devotes part of a chapter to research that has been done on schizophrenic and autistic patients who saw resolution of delusions and hallucinations as well as improvement in social skills simply with diet changes. I have experienced this. Without gluten, I feel a total sense of quick-firing within my brain, the ability to adapt easily, and the ability to find words efficiently. If I'm accidentally exposed to gluten, my brain turns to what feels like sludge. It processes much more slowly, and overall I feel like I've been drinking—and it even can take me a few days to recover.

Individuals with gluten sensitivity and celiac disease have even been found to have neurological symptoms other than brain fog (Hadjivassiliou et al. 2010). These symptoms include anxiety, depression, autism, attention deficit/hyperactivity disorder (ADHD), ataxia, and seizure disorders. Other neurological conditions include peripheral neuropathy, inflammatory myopathies, headaches, and even gluten encephalopathy (Jackson et al. 2012).

Because of the neurological symptoms that foods can cause, I've also seen patients sleep better—their insomnia resolves when they change their diet. It's been reported that even autistic children can improve once the inflammatory triggers are removed. In *Wheat Belly*, Davis writes that, "People who remove wheat from their diet typically report improved mood, fewer mood swings, improved ability to concentrate, and deeper sleep within just days to weeks of their last bite of a bagel or lasagna." Interestingly, people often crave exactly what they should *not* be eating. I found one patient—a fifty-year-old man who consumed three glasses of milk daily for nearly his entire life—to be severely intolerant to milk. His cravings for and addiction to milk made it difficult for him to get past the withdrawal stage. When he did, the cravings finally subsided.

His experience is similar to that of people trying to go sugar-free. Many patients crave and withdraw from sugar until it is entirely out of their system, and then their cravings resolve.

Patients often ask me how strict they need to be in avoiding the foods they react to. As a good friend, Joseph Collins, ND, RN, once told me, "Can you be just a little bit pregnant? No. Similarly, you either have food sensitivities, or you don't." In other words, you should 100 percent avoid the foods you reacted to, at least for a short period of time, though it can take months or years for the gastrointestinal lining to truly heal.

I recommend patients be tested yearly for food sensitivities. Sometimes we only see minor reductions in major reactions. As patients change their diets, they often cling to new foods they hadn't previously been eating and may encounter new sensitivities. Repeat tests help bring to light any new intolerances.

I recommend patients be tested yearly for food sensitivities.

Histamine Intolerance

Some patients flush in the face after eating certain foods or even after consuming alcohol. For instance, a patient may not test positive to avocado from an IgG standpoint, but if they become itchy or flush after eating it, they should still avoid it. Remember, the reaction could be separate from IgG. It could even be an IgE reaction. If food testing doesn't show any reaction, I question whether there's a poor immune system—maybe a low total IgA, or possibly a histamine intolerance.

Histamine is a chemical involved in regulating physiological functions—such as digestion in the gut—as well as in immune responses, and can also act as a neurotransmitter. Histamine triggers the inflammatory response. It is produced by basophils and by mast cells found in connective tissues, and is released in response to foreign pathogens. "Histamine causes your blood vessels to swell, or dilate, so that your white blood cells can quickly find and attack the infection or problem. The histamine buildup is what gives you a headache and leaves you feeling flushed, itchy and miserable. This is part of the body's natural immune response, but if you don't break down histamine properly, you could develop what we call histamine intolerance" (Myers 2013).

In the body, histamine must be stored or broken down by an enzyme. Histamine in the central nervous system is broken down primarily by histamine N-methyltransferase (HMT), while histamine in the digestive tract is broken down primarily by diamine oxidase (DAO). If you're deficient in DAO, you are at a greater likelihood to have symptoms of histamine intolerance.

SYMPTOMS OF HISTAMINE INTOLERANCE

- Headaches
- Migraines
- Difficulty falling asleep
- Easily aroused from sleep
- Vertigo or dizziness
- High blood pressure
- Flushing
- Anxiety
- Fatigue
- Elevated heart rates
- Difficulty regulating
- Body temperature
- Difficulty breathing
- Nausea or vomiting
- Abdominal cramps
- Nasal congestion
- Sneezing
- Itching and hives
- Abnormal menstrual cycle
- Tissue swelling

CAUSES OF HIGH HISTAMINE LEVELS

- Leaky gut
- IgE allergies to the environment or food
- Diet high in histamine-rich foods
- Fermented alcohol like wine, champagne, and beer
- Small intestine bacterial overgrowth (SIBO)
- Diamine oxidase (DAO) deficiency

Foods that either naturally contain histamine or block the enzyme that breaks it down (diamine oxidase) can cause symptoms in many patients.

The following is a list of histamine-rich and histamine-releasing foods that patients can avoid if they suspect histamine is causing problems:

HISTAMINE-RICH FOODS

- Fermented alcoholic beverages, especially wine, champagne and beer
- Fermented foods: sauerkraut, vinegar, soy sauce, kefir, yogurt, kombucha, etc
- Vinegar-containing foods: pickles, mayonnaise, olives
- Cured meats: bacon, salami, pepperoni, luncheon meats and hot dogs
- Soured foods: sour cream, sour milk, buttermilk, soured bread, etc
- Dried fruit: apricots, prunes, dates, figs, raisins
- Most citrus fruits
- Aged cheese including goat cheese
- Nuts: walnuts, cashews, and peanuts
- Vegetables: avocados, eggplant, spinach, and tomatoes
- Smoked fish and certain species of fish: mackerel, mahi-mahi, tuna, anchovies, sardines

HISTAMINE-RELEASING FOODS

- Alcohol
- Bananas
- Chocolate
- Cow's Milk
- Nuts
- Papaya
- Pineapple
- Shellfish
- Strawberries
- Tomatoes
- Wheat Germ
- Many artificial preservatives and dyes

In my own experience, I noticed my flushing greatly reduced after I went on a strictly gluten-free diet. Why? Gluten blocks DAO. Very interestingly, although one might think that histamine-blocking medication would help prevent histamine intolerance, these medications can actually deplete DAO levels in your body, worsening the issue. Other medications that can deplete DAO include nonsteroidal anti-inflammatory drugs (NSAIDs), antidepressants, antihistamines, histamine blockers, immune modulators, and antiarrhythmics (Myers 2013). Foods that block DAO include alcohol, energy drinks, and black and green teas. Low DAO can also be caused by gluten intolerance, leaky gut, SIBO, inflammatory diseases of the bowels, and genetics.

CAUSES OF LOW DAO

Gluten intolerance and sensitivity

Leaky gut

SIBO

DAO-blocking foods: alcohol, energy drinks, and tea

Genetic mutations (common in people of Asian descent)

Inflammation from Crohn's, ulcerative colitis, and inflammatory bowel disease

Medications:
Non-steroidal, anti-inflammatory drugs (ibuprofen, aspirin)

Antidepressants (Cymbalta, Effexor, Prozac, Zoloft)

Immune modulators (Humira, Enbrel, Plaquenil)

Antiarrhythmics (propanolol, metaprolol, Cardizem, Norvasc)

Antihistamines (Allegra, Zyrtec, Benadryl)

Histamine (H2) blockers (Tagamet, Pepcid, Zantac)

DAO-BLOCKING FOODS

Alcohol

Energy drinks

Black and green tea

If you think you may have histamine intolerance, get tested. Dunwoody Labs in Dunwoody, Georgia, can test you for histamine and DAO levels. A high ratio of histamine/DAO indicates that you are ingesting too much histamine and that you don't have enough DAO to break it down.

Also, try eliminating high-histamine foods for thirty days and reintroducing them one at a time, monitoring how you feel. Try taking DAO with meals. This may give you a glimpse into the issues, and, if your symptoms resolve, you could have low DAO. You may have taken an antihistamine or histamine blocker if you've suffered from seasonal allergies. Common names for these drugs are Allegra, Zyrtec, and even Benadryl. Find out if you have gluten sensitivity or SIBO and get off drugs that can reduce DAO.

If you struggle with histamine intolerance, then what foods can you eat? Here's a list of low-histamine foods that should be safer options.

LOW-HISTAMINE FOODS

Meat and poultry, freshly cooked, fresh or frozen

Freshly cooked fish (freshly caught only—no frozen)

Eggs

Pure peanut butter

Fresh vegetables, except those listed as histamine-rich (spinach, tomatoes, avocados, and eggplant)

Fresh fruits such as apple, watermelon, cantaloupe, grapes, mango, pear, and kiwi

Almond, coconut, rice, hemp milk, and other dairy substitutes

Gluten-free grains such as rice and quinoa

Olive oil and coconut oil for cooking

Leafy herbs for flavor

Herbal teas

The Low Histamine Chef, Jasmina Ykelenstam, at lowhistaminechef.com, and the mindbodygreen.com website, are two excellent resources for people dealing with histamine issues.

Still not sure if you have food sensitivities? Visit www.yourlongevityblueprint.com and fill out a symptom

questionnaire on food sensitivities, histamine intolerance, and even yeast overgrowth.

Often, I've found that patients who learn of their food sensitivities or food intolerances do not know where to start for removal. They are unaware of what food substitutes are available.

At our clinic, we have all our patients with food sensitivities meet with our health coach, who provides them handouts with the substitutions and helps guide them on a gut-healing protocol, which I'll share in the pages ahead. I do advise that you learn from an experienced health coach or nutritionist.

Many of our patients enjoy a paleo-like diet as well, also known as the hunter-gatherer diet. This diet naturally removes many of the top highly allergenic foods. It is high in saturated fats, moderately high in animal protein, and low in carbs. There are hundreds of excellent paleo guides online. I recommend Paleo Chef, and Paleo Mom.

Use the following lists to help you avoid gluten, eggs, and dairy—the most common food sensitivities—if you are trying an elimination diet or have already been tested.

FOODS/PRODUCTS CONTAINING **GLUTEN**

Wheat	Spelt	Croutons
Barley	Malt	Crackers
Rye	Breads	Sauces and Gravies
Oats	Pasta and Noodles	Tortillas
Semolina	Pastries	Beer

You may be surprised to learn that the glue on envelopes contains gluten. I found that out the hard way. I licked a huge stack of thank-you notes and felt sick immediately! Even some cosmetics, such as lipsticks, contain gluten. Once, on a trip in Galena, Illinois, I purchased a bubble bath, and was eager to get back to our cottage to take a relaxing bath until I discovered the main ingredient in the product was "wheat protein."

When I first started my gluten-free lifestyle I thought rice cereal was gluten-free, since it was made out of rice. However, you absolutely *must* read labels. Many rice cereals, if not marked gluten-free, contain "malt," which has gluten. I was also surprised to learn that many over-the-counter (OTC) medications contain gluten or lactose (milk sugar). I have several patients on thyroid medications who needed to be gluten-free based on their food testing and their autoimmune thyroid condition, yet their thyroid medication contained gluten. I now know what common medications contain and do not contain gluten, but I advise all patients to take the time to call their pharmacists on all their medications.

FOODS/PRODUCTS CONTAINING **EGGS**

Baked goods	Custards	Dressings
Pasta	Frosting	Root beer
Marshmallows	Puddings	Specialty coffee drinks
Mayonnaise	Sauces	Breaded dishes

FOODS/PRODUCTS CONTAINING **DAIRY**

Whey	Goat's milk products	Egg replacers
Casein	Scrambled Eggs	Lunch meats
Cow's milk products: cheese, butter, yogurt, cream, and ice cream	Mashed/scalloped dishes	Instant cocoa preparations
	Hot dogs	Select non-dairy substitutes

This means that protein powders and even some protein bars that state they are dairy-free are *not* dairy-free, because they contain whey or casein. My favorite protein powders that we carry at our clinic are collagen, bone broth, hemp, hydrolyzed organic beef, rice, pea, and potato protein. All are gluten-, dairy-, and egg-free.

Some of my favorite resources for an allergen-friendly diet are Food Babe, Paleo Mom, Low Histamine Chef, and sometimes even Pinterest. Check out our clinic website, ihhclinic.com, for recipes and alternatives as well.

PHASE 1B: REMOVE GASTROINTESTINAL INFECTIONS

Now that I've discussed the importance of removing foods that you react to, let's discuss gastrointestinal infections.

Yeast or Candida

Several of my patients have struggled with yeast overgrowth. A yeast infection is simply an infection of a fungus such as candida, though I have found several other types of yeast infections in my patients. For simplicity, I will stick to discussing candida and will use the term "yeast." These infections can inhabit the gut, skin, vagina, and genitourinary tract.

Sometimes the symptoms are not as obvious to the patient as to the clinician. For instance, unlike a persistent vaginal yeast infection, brain fog may not alert the patient that they are susceptible to or have yeast overgrowth. But, as a clinician, I commonly see the combination of bloating, brain fog, weight gain, fatigue, and frequent yeast infections—especially in patients who have been given antibiotics—which raises my suspicion of yeast overgrowth. Antibiotics are given for ear infections, sinus infections, bladder infections, and acne, setting the stage for yeast overgrowth. It's important to have a strong gastrointestinal foundation prior to taking antibiotics so that yeast won't flair.

SYMPTOMS OF YEAST SENSITIVITY OR OVERGROWTH

Bloating	Bad breath
Brain fog	Chronic sinus infections
Weight gain	Frequent vaginal yeast infections
Fatigue	Skin and nail infections

Patients who take one round of antibiotics every five years do not always have their good bacteria wiped out by the medication. On the other hand, patients who take two or three courses of antibiotics during the winter for sinus infections or other upper respiratory infections—or those patients who have taken antibiotics for acne daily for years on end—are more susceptible to having their gut bacteria affected. In my opinion, providers who prescribe antibiotics for patients should also always discuss the long-term risks of that medication—being yeast overgrowth. Patients often don't care, as they are signing up for the short-term benefits of, say, acne improvement, but it may make them think twice if the side effects are discussed in advance—especially since chronic yeast overgrowth can lead to chronic fatigue syndrome, which can be debilitating.

Just as medical providers typically do not discuss side effects when they prescribe antibiotics, they also do not prescribe nutrients to replace those that prescription drugs often deplete. For instance, if a woman is prescribed birth control, she should also be prescribed a B complex, since birth control depletes the body of B vitamins. Similarly, if a patient is prescribed a statin, or cholesterol-lowering medication, he or she should be prescribed coenzyme Q10, a nutrient that statins rob the body of. Unfortunately, informing the patient about nutrient depletion caused by prescriptions is still not mainstream practice. (More on this topic in chapter 4.) In conventional medicine—remembering the carpenter-versus-fireman approach discussed earlier—patients are going to their physicians only in order to get their fire extinguished. Instead, the provider should be getting at the root cause of why the patient has acne, or any other symptom, in the first place, and not just have the patient take antibiotics for years at a time.

Other patients who are susceptible to yeast include those with uncontrolled diabetes, since sugar feeds yeast. People on steroids are also susceptible, because steroids suppress the immune system. Plus, steroids can increase blood glucose levels, which, again, feeds yeast. Patients who are already immunocompromised, such as those with cancer or AIDS, are more susceptible as well.

There are several ways to test for yeast. High baker's and brewer's yeast on IgG or IgA food testing suggests yeast sensitivity. This is an immune reaction similar to candida antibodies in the blood. These tests are looking at chronic delayed hypersensitivity reactions. Additionally, a comprehensive stool analysis is a better test for acute or current yeast overgrowth in the gut. The strength in stool testing is that many labs will offer a culture and sensitivity, meaning that if there is yeast overgrowth, the lab will reveal which antifungal medications and which botanical options the yeast is sensitive to and which options the yeast is resistant to. This type of test is commonly run for urinary tract infections, but not so commonly used for patients with yeast symptoms.

Over the years, I have had several patients' stool testing show me that their particular persistent strain of yeast was actually resistant to the commonly prescribed medication fluconazole (Diflucan), or even Nystatin. However, their provider was unaware of this, and had continued to prescribe them those medications for years. There is a time and place for using medications like Diflucan, however, Diflucan can be very hard on the liver. Similarly, I've had patients consume antifungals that they have read on the internet are beneficial, yet their particular testing showed that their yeast was resistant to the agents they were using. Thorough testing helps identify which agents should or should not be used with these patients for the patient's ultimate success.

It's interesting that it's often assumed that if a patient has yeast on their stool test, they must have gastrointestinal symptoms (GI), but in fact the patient doesn't have to have any GI symptoms. In Jacob Teitelbaum's book, *From Fatigue to Fantastic*, he discusses how nearly all his patients with chronic fatigue and fibromyalgia (not GI symptoms) have chronic yeast (Teitelbaum 2007).

One of the worst cases of candida I've seen was a middle-aged woman. She had been taking Diflucan twice weekly for years, which was still not controlling a rash in her axilla (underarm) area. It took months of the daily highest dose of Diflucan, a natural antifungal protocol, and major dietary changes to finally eradicate it.

Symptoms of candida can manifest on various body locations, and can include a rash, reddened or white flaking or scaling, cracks in the skin, soreness, and redness. Many individuals are familiar with diaper rash seen in a baby, or athlete's foot in an adult. These are both due to yeast. Athlete's foot (tinea pedis) is the yeast (fungal) infection that usually begins between the toes. It can occur in people whose feet have become very moist or sweaty while confined within tight-fitting shoes. These patients typically notice red and white scaling and experience intense itching. Women may experience this same rash between or below their breasts, as that is also a location where moisture can collect. Yeast likes to grow in deep, dark, moist places like the sinus cavities and vagina. Again, individuals with diabetes are at a higher risk for yeast, as sugar feeds yeast. Oftentimes, part of truly getting yeast under control involves controlling diabetes.

Cracks on the corner of the mouth are commonly caused by yeast as well. If an obvious rash isn't noted, other physical symptoms suggesting yeast overgrowth may still be present, like fungus on the toenails, or white/yellow plaque on the tongue. During a physical exam, I always assess my patient's oral cavity, corners of the mouth, tongue, and nails.

Another challenge for several of my patients with chronic yeast is that their symptoms are never entirely eradicated until their partner is also treated for yeast. Incidentally the husband of one of my patients came with her to her follow-up appointment after she finished an antifungal protocol. Although her symptoms had improved, she still noticed symptoms flared after intercourse. Since her husband was present at the appointment, I looked at his tongue, which I found to be thickly coated with yeast. He didn't have any noted penile discharge to report. However, his tongue suggested he may have systemic yeast. I then was able to explain to both of them that yeast would not be entirely eradicated until both of them were properly treated.

How do you know if you have a yeast or other infection? Test! I commonly use Genova Diagnostics GI Effects 2200 panel with my patients. Several other functional medicine labs offer similar testing. I have also used Doctor's Data. A three-day test is superior to a one-day test, as a one-day test could miss an infection. The stool test includes a bacterial and mycological culture, which demonstrates the presence of specific beneficial and pathological organisms. Parasitology also looks for markers for pathogens like *Campylobacter, Clostridium difficile, Escherichia coli,* and *Helicobacter pylori* stool antigen.

One of my first severe yeast cases was a sixty-six-year-old woman who had a long history of irritable bowel syndrome, and who found herself incredibly tired—experiencing bloating, reflux, and unquenchable hunger. Testing revealed several food intolerances and significant yeast overgrowth.

Testing: For this patient, I tested for yeast in two ways—serum (blood) candida IgA and IgG. Both delivered positive results. Additionally, I ordered Genova's GI Effects stool test. Interestingly, the patient had 4+ candida glabrata; 4+ is the highest level that Genova registers.

Treatment options: Because the test ordered on her provided a sensitivity report, I knew how to treat her. Her yeast wasn't sensitive to Diflucan, but it was sensitive to Nystatin as well as several natural botanical treatment options including berberine, caprylic acid, garlic, undecylenic acid, and uva ursi.

Her treatment protocol heavily emphasized dietary changes to inhibit feeding yeast, an essential first step for successful eradication. *The Body Ecology Diet,* by Donna Gates, and *The Yeast Connection Handbook*, by William G. Crook, MD, heavily discusses these necessary diet changes. Secondly, we treated her with Nystatin, working up in potency and frequency to several times a day for months. Upon retesting, the yeast had reduced from 4+ to 2+, which was still too high. We then reduced the medication to once daily and started her on the natural antifungals.

> **My favorite Longevity Blueprint (LB) product for yeast is our Advanced Yeast Complex. To learn more, visit yourlongevityblueprint.com.**

The reason the medications or supplements should be started slowly and then increased is to prevent a Herxheimer reaction. This is an immune system reaction to the toxins (endotoxins) that are released when large amounts of pathogens are being killed off and the body does not eliminate the toxins quickly enough. I've experienced this when I tried my own protocol. Simply put, I felt like I had the flu; I had nausea, aches and pains, and headaches. The symptoms only lasted a weekend, and were gone by Monday. These nasty symptoms are actually a good thing—a response indicating the body is ridding itself of toxins. But those terrible symptoms can usually be reduced by slowly working into a protocol instead of hitting it hard at the beginning. If the reaction is too severe, cutting back on the dosage or frequency of use can be very helpful in lessening symptoms, by allowing the healing process to continue.

Another important part of treating yeast is introducing enough good bacteria to keep the yeast at bay. I use various probiotics for this. Some patients with yeast issues can tolerate *Saccharomyces boulardii* (SB), which is a beneficial yeast, while others cannot. If they can tolerate SB, I use LB's Probiotic Complex with seven strains plus SB. If they cannot tolerate SB, I use Advanced Probiotic without SB.

Parasites

Parasites are organisms that can live in the human intestine, where they feed on nutrients and disrupt the body's systems. Common symptoms of parasites are nausea, vomiting, abdominal pain, excessive and persistent diarrhea, mucus, and blood in stools. However, I have seen patients experience other symptoms, such as fatigue and headaches, without having the commonly associated severe diarrhea. Parasites are common from drinking untreated water. I have patients who have parasites after returning from traveling to other countries, and other patients who don't initially have symptoms but who develop with them months down the road. I also see parasite cases more commonly in patients who raise or work with animals, specifically horses. These details illustrate why a thorough medical history is so important.

Testing: The benefit of running a parasite test through a larger lab is that the lab can run a microscopic examination for ova (eggs) and parasites, which is the gold standard. They can also run an enzyme immune assay (EIA). The most common parasites I have seen in my functional medicine practice are *Blactocystis hominis, Cryptosporidium, Dientamoeba fragilis, Entamoeba histolytica,* and *Giardia lamblia.*

Treatment options: I have used botanical options to help treat parasites; however, they are sometimes not strong enough. Pharmaceutical treatment options include metronidazole (flagyl), nitazoxanide, and iodoquinol.

Helicobacter pylori (H. pylori)

H. pylori is commonly known for causing gastritis, duodenal, and peptic ulcer disease, and it can also eventually lead to gastric cancer (lymphoma). It is estimated that up to 40 percent of US adults are affected; however, many remain asymptomatic. The many symptoms of *H. pylori* include excessive burping, bloating, nausea, vomiting, loss of appetite, unexplained weight loss, and foul breath.

Testing: Blood and stool tests that measure specific *H. pylori* IgG antibodies can determine if a person has been infected.

Treatment options: Conventional treatment involves a proton pump inhibitor, as well as antibiotics. Although I do not encourage long-term use of proton pump inhibitors (reflux medications), I do believe there is a time and place for short-term usage.

Many patients who've suffered from *H. pylori*, and who've taken countless antibiotics, prefer to avoid drug dependency. Luckily, there are natural options to help eradicate this infection. The most popular LB product I use is Pylori Essentials, formulated to help heal the stomach lining. It contains zinc carnosine (a zinc complex of L-carnosine approved in Japan since 1994 for its use in stomach health), mastic gum (traditionally used to protect the stomach lining), bismuth citrate (used to promote normal bacterial growth, and to soothe gastric and mucosal lining), and, finally, a natural antibacterial compound, berberine sulfate (Ortho Molecular).

Clostridium difficile (C. difficile)

Once you've smelled the unpleasant *Clostridium difficile* (*C. difficile* or *C. diff*), you will never forget it. Due to numerous rounds of antibiotics often given to a patient in the hospital, patients can develop the *C. diff* colonization that can lead to severe abdominal pain, cramping, fever, watery diarrhea, nausea, and loss of appetite. Interestingly, the treatment is more antibiotics, which eventually can lead to some antibiotic resistance. Vancomycin or metronidazole are the common antibiotic treatments; however, herbal agents like berberine and oregano have been shown to be beneficial. I also often have patients use *Saccharomyces boulardii* (SB), as well as silver with aloe vera as the delivery agent. Even Mayo Clinic suggests *Saccharomyces boulardii* for preventing and treating *C. diff* (Mayo 2016). For those who are prone to this condition, I always recommend this organism when they're on antibiotics, staggering it so that it is taken a few hours before or after the antibiotics. Also, several of my patients take this daily as part of their maintenance probiotic regimen.

Typically, the symptoms of *C. diff* are so severe that patients are already in the hospital, or were seen in urgent care, immediately after the symptoms started to occur. In my practice, I commonly see recurrent infections. I had one patient around twenty-six years old who had already suffered with *C. diff* three times, and who was worried it had returned again, when she came to my clinic.

PACKING SLIP

Bay State Books

111-5340405-4636209

6177509221
1245 Providence HWY
suite 1
Sharon, MA 02067

SHIP TO:

CRAIG CARROLL
314282940288040
192 EARL DR
TWIN FALLS, ID 83301-7613
United States

VIA:

Order Number:
Order Date: 01/28/2022
Shipping Method: Standard Std US D2D Dom

SKU	QTY	TITLE	TOTAL
BSM.23VU	1	Your Longevity Blueprint: Building A Healthier Body Through Functional Medicine [Paperback] [2017] Gray, Stephanie	10.39

Order Total: 11.01

Special Instructions:

#164080 DSC p42374361o164080_T47-OSMDOM-_898- 1/2

Testing: She was tested in two ways. I ordered the *C. diff* sample to a local lab and also sent out the sample to Genova for a more comprehensive assessment. I didn't want to miss a positive. Her test was positive through both labs.

Treatment options: This particular patient did not want to take antibiotics, for fear that she would develop either worsening symptoms or a vaginal yeast infection. Instead, I treated her with twenty billion colony-forming units (CFUs) of *Saccharomyces boulardii* (SB), as well as with silver hydrosol and aloe vera three times daily. Within two weeks, she was starting to feel back to normal.

For these recurrent cases, I suggest testing the stool a few times per year to verify total eradication and to assess the gastrointestinal microbiome. Our LB supplement with SB used to treat *C. diff* is called Beneficial Yeast.

SIBO

A typical stool test looks at what is happening in the large intestine, otherwise known as the colon. It is very difficult to detect what is happening in the small intestine (SI), yet infections can occur there, too. I've had patients whose stool tests were uniquely optimal, and yet they were experiencing bloating or diarrhea. In these cases, specifically when patients have more upper gastrointestinal symptoms versus lower symptoms, or when the lower (colon) stool test is negative, it is important to test for small intestinal bacterial overgrowth (SIBO).

SIBO is a chronic infection of the small intestine from bacteria that normally live in the gastrointestinal tract but have abnormally overgrown in a location not meant for so many bacteria. Unfortunately, these bacteria can interfere with normal digestion and absorption, and can also contribute to leaky gut.

Common presenting symptoms for SIBO include upper gastrointestinal fullness, bloating, an urge to burp or belch, trouble swallowing, and/or fullness in the throat. Some people also experience abdominal pains and irregular bowels. However, some have normal bowels, as in my case. I had no bowel problems per se, yet I was so full of gas and the constant need to burp that I was always uncomfortable and short of breath.

Testing: Unfortunately, there is no perfect test for SIBO, since it's difficult to access the middle portion of the small intestine.

An upper endoscopy only allows access to the top portion of the small intestine, and a colonoscopy only allows access to the end portion. Therefore, the most commonly used test is a breath test. The test involves the patient undergoing a one- or two-day preparatory diet to remove most of the food in the intestine that feeds bacteria. The patient then drinks a sugar solution consisting of glucose or lactulose. So, since the food has been removed and lactulose cannot be digested or absorbed except by bacteria, once the patient consumes the sugar solution their body will create gas. The test measures hydrogen and methane gasses generated over the next two to three hours to determine whether there is an overgrowth (SIBO Info).

Patients can often order these test kits online and perform the breath testing in their home. However, the lactulose must be ordered through a provider, since it requires a prescription.

Treatment options: Treatment is primarily aimed at reducing the bacteria level. This can be done with antibiotics like metronidazole (Flagyl), however this drug tends to cause more vaginal yeast infections in my patients. Other, superior options exist. The preferred drug is rifaximin (Xifaxan), although neomycin may also be used. These are preferred because they are almost completely nonabsorbable, which means they stay in the intestines, where they have a local action, rather than systemic (body-wide) side effects such as yeast infection. The Xifaxan dosage I use the most is 550 mg three times daily (TID) for ten to fourteen days.

Many patients prefer a more natural approach, or have already tried antibiotics and failed, or are not comfortable having to take antibiotics every year. Some botanicals that can be effective in treating SIBO include allicin from garlic (high potency), oregano, and berberine. I use a similar product for treatment of SIBO, yeast, and bacteria called Advanced Yeast Complex.

I have also used a silver/aloe vera combination for some cases. Silver is antibacterial, and, when taken on an empty stomach with a delivery agent such as aloe vera, it is thought to make it past the stomach acid into the SI to kill off bacteria. This protocol involves taking the silver three times daily on an empty stomach for as long as eight weeks. These patients also need to focus on healing the gut lining, removing any food intolerances, and focusing on the fourth R, Repair (which I discuss more in detail later in this chapter).

There are several supplements that can help reduce gas associated with this condition. LB Peppermint Oil contains peppermint, fennel, and ginger. This combination helps to relax the GI muscles, causing fewer spasms. It also helps to reduce gas and indigestion.

Activated charcoal can also be used to help absorb gas. It can be taken every few hours, but can cause darkened stools and constipation. It's a highly absorbent material with millions of pores to capture unwanted materials. It has a negative charge that binds positively charged toxins and gas to be excreted out of the body (bulletproof.com 2017).

Diets are also incredibly important in these cases. The SIBO treatment diets are the specific carbohydrate diet (SCD), the gut and psychology syndrome diet (GAPS Diet, discussed in-depth in the Campbell-McBride book *Gut and Psychology Syndrome*), and the low FODMAP diet (LFD). You can also use a combination of these diets.

FODMAPs are defined as a collection of short-chain carbohydrates and sugar alcohols found in foods naturally or as additives. FODMAPs include fructose (when in excess of glucose), fructans, galacto-oligosaccharides (GOS), and lactose and polyols (such as sorbitol and mannitol).

Removing FODMAP foods aims at reducing carbs, sugar, and food sources to bacteria.

WHAT DOES **FODMAP** STAND FOR?

F FERMENTABLE
Broken down (eaten/fermented) by bacteria in the large bowel

O OLIGOSACCHARIDES
Molecules made up of individual sugars joined together in a chain

D DISACCHARIDES
Double sugar molecule

M MONOSACCHARIDES
Single-sugar molecule

A AND

P POLYOLS
Sugar alcohols

THE DIET

ALLOWED
Meat/fish/poultry, eggs, some beans, lactose-free dairy, non-starchy vegetables, ripe fruit, nuts/seeds, honey, and saccharine.

NOT ALLOWED
Grains, starchy vegetables, lactose, some beans, any sweeteners other than honey, saccharine, and occasional stevia.

Initially cooked vegetables, cooked ripe fruit, no beans, and very little nuts are recommended.

Initially, it's recommended to eat cooked vegetables, cooked ripe fruit, no beans, and very few nuts. For more information on this diet, visit www.siboinfo.com.

Several of my patients with SIBO have unfortunately experienced refractory disease, meaning the symptoms keep returning every few months. Unfortunately I know this far too well, as I have also experienced SIBO. These patients should be placed on a protocol to help prevent the relapses. The protocol typically includes long-term botanicals and the low FODMAP diet, although over time it can usually be adjusted to be less strict.

Some providers are experimenting with **biofilm busters** for these patients as well. Biofilms are a group of microorganisms that stick to each other, creating a self-produced matrix or slime, which can make it difficult for antibiotics to break through. Thus, many antibiotics are now given with biofilm busters. Biocidin is the common name for a popular biofilm-busting product. I've commonly seen these used for Lyme infections, but they are also starting to be used in SIBO treatment as well.

One particularly interesting case was a thirty-one-year-old man, Michael, who came to my clinic for a third opinion. He reported abdominal pains and daily nausea, stating that he'd had indigestion since he was eighteen. He tested positive for fructose intolerance, and a previous allergist had told him he had a "mild dairy allergy." All of his additional testing—blood work, gallbladder ultrasound, abdominal computed tomography (CT), and colonoscopy—were normal. He had been placed on a proton pump inhibitor, omeprazole. One provider had prescribed a medication called Bentyl, which was supposed to reduce spasms. However, Michael felt the medication made his symptoms worsen. He also did not tolerate probiotics well, and they worsened his symptoms. He had lost over twenty pounds, likely due to malabsorption of nutrients. We tested him for food sensitivities and found that his gluten levels were very high. His SIBO testing was positive, and his stool test showed very high fat levels, indicating that he was not absorbing his fats, which commonly occurs in those with SIBO.

His treatment involved rifaximin (Xifaxan) along with a strict gluten-free diet. He was already on a low FODMAP diet due to the known fructose intolerance. He was also placed on ox bile with fatty meals. After treating the infection, we were able to slowly wean him off his proton pump inhibitor, and his nausea reduced; he was able to gain weight back. He was a classic case of undetected and untreated SIBO and food sensitivities, and I'm happy to report that he is now feeling and functioning much more optimally.

Fructose Intolerance

There can be overlap between symptoms of SIBO and fructose intolerance, and typically I test patients for both concurrently. What is fructose intolerance? According to the Mayo Clinic, "Fructose is a sugar found naturally in fruits, fruit juices, some vegetables, and honey. Fructose is also a basic component in table sugar (sucrose), and high-fructose corn syrup is used to sweeten many processed foods and beverages. When your digestive system doesn't absorb fructose properly, it can cause abdominal pain, diarrhea, and gas" (Mayo 2016). The main symptoms are bloating, belching, distension, gas, abdominal pain, and diarrhea (Fedewa and Rao 2015).

Testing: Similar to SIBO breath testing.

Treatment: The Mayo Clinic reports that no pharmaceutical treatment for fructose intolerance exists, "although some individuals believe digestive enzymes may help some" (Mayo 2016). Mayo suggests that people with fructose intolerance "should limit high-fructose foods, such as juices, apples, grapes, watermelon, asparagus, peas, and zucchini" (Mayo 2016). They add that "lower fructose foods—such as bananas, blueberries, strawberries, carrots, avocados, green beans, and lettuce—may be tolerated in limited quantities with meals."

My recommendation? Read product labels carefully and avoid foods containing:

- fructose and high-fructose corn syrup
- natural sugars such as honey, agave syrup, maple syrup, molasses, and palm or coconut sugar
- sorghum

Sadly, I've experienced SIBO and fructose intolerance, too. I suffered from a tremendous need to belch, and what I describe as air trapping, also causing shortness of breath. Food testing and a gluten-free diet weren't enough to heal my gut (although gluten was likely the primary cause). Some gas-producing foods didn't show up on the food sensitivity test, because I didn't mount an immune response to them. To heal, I had to treat SIBO and avoid both my IgG reactions and high FODMAP foods. A gastroenterologist placed me on a proton pump inhibitor (PPI), typically used for heartburn, and took a wait-and-see approach. I took the medication out of desperation, but it didn't help. I ended up going to urgent care the night before flying to Mexico for a family wedding. That doctor recommended I double the reflux medication as well as start Bentyl to help reduce spasms in my throat. He didn't even think about trying to explore the root cause of the problem. That night I looked up contraindications for Bentyl and found reflux—the reason I was prescribed the PPI. I decided I'd be better off without it, so I asked my family doctor's opinion and she agreed that it should not have been prescribed for me. I quit taking it altogether. Sadly, taking the PPI increased my risk for SIBO, as did my history of Ibuprofen use.

Lactose Intolerance

Lactose intolerance may be the most common and well-known genetic disease in the world. Many individuals are aware of their lactose intolerance, because they have abdominal pain, distension, and terrible-smelling gas after eating yogurt, milk, or ice cream. This is related to a lactase deficiency.

Lactose intolerance is different from a dairy sensitivity. Individuals with this intolerance don't make the enzyme lactase that breaks down the milk sugar lactose, which is why they get bloated and gassy. Having a dairy sensitivity could make you gassy but could also cause acne, skin issues, and even headaches or fatigue. Individuals with lactose intolerance should still be tested for dairy sensitivity, as taking lactase enzyme will not resolve the immune response.

Testing: The aforementioned hydrogen breath test can also assess for lactose intolerance. However, the breath test can register a false positive if the patient also has SIBO.

Treatment: Treatment is most successful with the combination of diet, enzymes (such as lactase), and probiotics. These patients also benefit from the diets for SIBO and fructose intolerance (a low FODMAP diet).

In my experience, patients usually don't have only fructose or lactose intolerance. They usually also have other food sensitivities, and, again, simply taking a lactase pill won't resolve those. As mentioned in the SIBO case study, Michael knew he had fructose intolerance, but he also needed to be tested for food sensitivities and GI infections.

After removing the food sensitivities and treating the GI infections, you must move on to the next four phases to truly heal your gut: replace, reinoculate, repair, and rebalance.

PHASE 2: REPLACE

The second R, **Replace**, specifically refers to improving and replacing bile, acid, and enzymes to help facilitate better digestion.

Digestion and Maldigestion

Digestion starts with the act of chewing. Think of your teeth as the blades of a food processor breaking down food into chunks before swallowing. The salivary glands in your mouth secrete different enzymes (amylases) to start breaking down the food. It's very important to chew thoroughly to get this process started.

Experts suggest chewing your food at least twenty times. It's also important to avoid having a dry mouth, which, as you can imagine, lacks these enzymes. If you can't chew well, pureeing food can help with digestion. It's also important to avoid drinking too much water with meals, since that can dilute the mouth of necessary enzymes.

Swallowed food travels down the long esophagus tube into the **stomach**. That is where carbohydrate digestion starts. Pepsin, trypsin, chymotrypsin, and hydrochloric acid are secreted to help digest proteins. This process can take hours. The stomach continues to churn your food, and it becomes mixed into a solution called chyme, which then travels to the **small intestine**.

That's where enzymes like lipase and bile—secreted from the **pancreas** and the **gallbladder**, respectfully—assist with fat digestion. Starches are broken down into simple sugars, fats are broken down into fatty acids and glycerine, and proteins are broken down into amino acids. The small intestine houses many bacteria, also known as the microbiome (these are important in the next step, Reinoculate). Absorption of nutrients should take place in the small intestine. Then the remaining food passes through a valve called the ileocecal valve into the large intestine, where it absorbs water and electrolytes and even gastric juices. That leaves you a semisolid bowel movement.

The **large intestine** also houses various bacteria. After the large intestine completes its job, the remaining waste is eliminated.

The **liver** is also vital to digestion. The blood from the intestinal tract goes through the liver, which then decides what nutrients to keep or toxins to excrete. The unwanted toxins leave the liver through the bile.

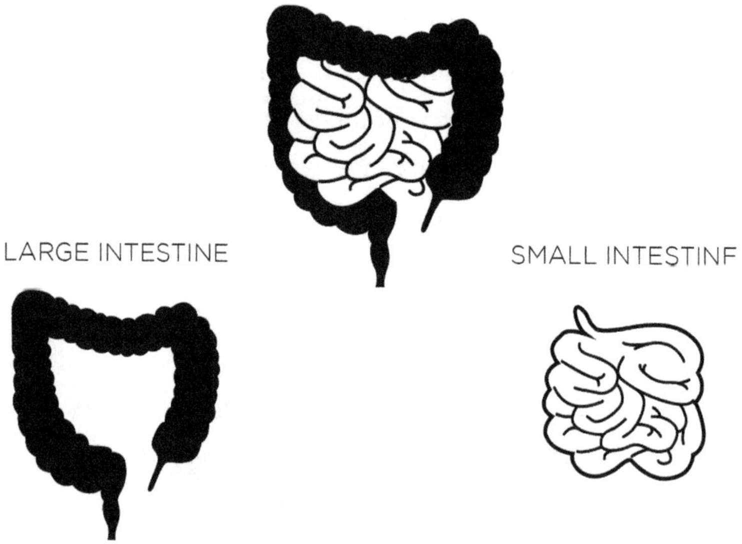

Without proper digestion, food literally rots inside the body. Putrefaction is a process in which proteins are not digested but instead are converted by intestinal bacteria into toxic substances, often smelling like sulfur. That can happen if you eat too much, don’t chew well, or are deficient in enzymes, hydrochloric acid (HCL), or bile. Carbohydrates can ferment, converting sugars to methane gas, alcohol, and acetaldehyde. You can often tell if this has occurred by the foul smell of your bowel movement (Wilson 2016).

The four takeaways from this summary of digestion are that you need saliva, enzymes, HCL, and bile. How do you know if you have enough enzymes, HCL, and bile? Test. I commonly find that patients not only have food sensitivities, but their comprehensive stool test also reveals digestion issues. The test mentioned previously for assessing for gut infections also shows many digestion and absorption markers.

One patient suffered with diarrhea daily since having her gallbladder removed. After a suggestion to take bile with fatty meals, her diarrhea nearly entirely resolved. Fecal fat, which is a marker of fat breakdown and absorption, can be tested in the stool. High fecal fat can indicate pancreatic insufficiency, bile salt insufficiency, low stomach acid, and SIBO. Fecal fat can also be high with intestinal parasites, other infections, excessive alcohol intake, use of NSAIDs, and even inflammatory bowel disease and other food intolerances. **Bile** helps with fat absorption. I thought bile might help this patient, since she no longer had her gallbladder; however, I still see patients who have their gall bladder (although it may not be functioning properly) who have high fat in their stools and need bile. Bile also helps to regulate pathogenic load, and therefore can be helpful in patients with GI infections. It is typically given with high-fat meals.

Protein in the stool can also be tested. Now, a high-protein diet can skew some results high. If the patient is not on a high-protein diet, and protein is found high in the stool, this suggests a need for more enzymes and stomach acid, also known as hydrochloric acid or **betain hydrochloride (HCL)**. As you age, your HCL levels drop. It is estimated that 30 percent of the elderly have low levels (Champagne 1989). Have you ever seen vertical ridges on the nails of the elderly? These suggest low stomach acid. The medical term for low stomach acid is hypochlorhydria. I see this even in young individuals, unfortunately, because they have been placed on acid-blocking medications, those proton pump inhibitors. Examples of some of these are omeprazole (Prilosec), esomeprazole (Nexium), lansoprazole (Prevacid), rabeprazole (AcipHex), pantoprazole (Protonix), and dexlansoprazole (Dexilant).

HCL is necessary to prevent GI infections; it helps kill bacteria. In fact, a common side effect listed on the package insert for medications like omeprazole is SIBO, as well as other gut infections. Unfortunately, this is precisely what I encountered in my own experience. Before I eliminated gluten from my diet, I was placed on omeprazole for heartburn, which led to SIBO. The root cause had been the gluten in the first place!

So, how do you know if you are absorbing the foods you eat and the supplements you take? A comprehensive stool test can provide insight. You also don't want to see undigested food in your stool. However, the best way to know is to also run a comprehensive nutritional evaluation, which is further discussed in chapter 4.

Many patients ask me if we can test them to see if they have low HCL. Although I currently do not offer this at my clinic, one available way to check for low HCL is with the Heidelberg stomach acid test. With this test, the individual swallows a capsule, which then records the pH in the stomach. However, this is the most invasive means of testing. If the stool test suggests they need it, or if symptoms suggest they are low, I place them on an HCL challenge. See our website, **www.yourlongevityblueprint.com**, for this handout.

A stool test can also look for pancreatic exocrine insufficiency, which is common when protein levels are high in the stool. This insufficiency can be treated by taking **pancreatic enzyme replace-**

ment. What are pancreatic digestive enzymes? These enzymes are responsible for the digestion of food and the absorption of nutrients into our bodies, followed by the elimination of the nonessential and toxic ingredients (Bohager 2009). In other words, enzymes convert our food into energy. Different enzymes help break down different proteins: proteases break down proteins, lipases break down lipids or fats, carbohydrases break down carbohydrates, and cellulases break down cellulose.

Different enzymes help break down different proteins: proteases break down proteins, lipases break down lipids or fats, carbohydrases break down carbohydrates, and cellulases break down cellulose.

One of the main ingredients in several digestive enzymes is bromelain, from pineapple. Several of my patients have pineapple sensitivities, so they require pineapple-free enzymes. We carry one enzyme with pineapple and one without.

Many patients try apple cider vinegar (ACV) as well, which can help with digestion. It has been thought to be a super food. This is a fermented beverage containing enzymes and probiotics. ACV has also been shown to increase bile products, as previously discussed. ACV contains the organic acid acetic acid, which can help with acid reflux. It has also been shown to improve metabolism, help with weight loss, reduce blood pressure, reduce blood sugar, and reduce cholesterol levels. One or two tablespoons can be consumed straight or in water before meals to improve digestion and improve absorption of nutrients from food. It can also be used in many homemade salad dressing recipes.

It's important to note that some patients with yeast sensitivity cannot tolerate vinegar, so they can't tolerate ACV.

Some experts advise not to drink any water or other liquids with meals, and only after fifteen minutes following meals. Eat slowly and relax while eating. Don't rush. Also, to improve your digestion, think about avoiding processed foods, and eat some raw foods—which are loaded with enzymes—each day. Minimize overcooking and microwaving.

The digestion process may be the most important process we have for our health. Obviously, sleep is important as well, but if we don't have healthy digestion, we simply don't have health. If your digestion is not optimal, you have options. Consider taking Longevity Blueprint digestive support products.

PHASE 3: REESTABLISH OR REINOCULATE

The third R in a gut-healing protocol stands for **Reestablishing**, or **Reinoculating**, your gut with good bacteria. Part of the theory that the large majority of our immune system lies in our gut will be explained in this section. The gastrointestinal microbiome is housed in the gut, and that is what needs to be reinoculated, or as I like to describe it, "repopulated," with good bacteria.

In the reinoculate phase, according to the Institute for Functional Medicine, a combination of **probiotics** and prebiotics are added slowly to allow the GI tract to adjust. What exactly are probiotics? They are beneficial living microorganisms that support health in both gastrointestinal and immune systems. Because hundreds of diverse microbial species (some good and some bad) pass daily through the gastrointestinal tract in a healthy digestive system, these microorganisms should coexist in a balanced harmony (Klaire Labs

2016). When they do not, bad things can happen, and disease can set in.

Many patients ask me if they can consume enough of certain foods to feed the good bacteria in the gut. Some foods can help, but the food sources aren't as high in these bacteria as the probiotics supplements that are available. Fermented foods include some cheeses, yogurt, sauerkraut, kefir, and kimchi. I also have patients who enjoy drinking fermented beverages like kombucha. Most of my patients need much higher doses of probiotics than are found in these foods, and many can't tolerate the prebiotics—more on this later.

Surprisingly, many individuals are totally unaware of what prebiotics and probiotics are. Nobel Laureate Ilya Mechnikov first discovered the health benefits of fermented foods like yogurt. He identified *Lactobacillus bulgaricus* as a strain potentially responsible for Bulgarians living long, healthy lives. In *The Probiotics Revolution: The Definitive Guide to Safe, Natural Health Solutions*, author Gary Huffnagle describes good bacteria as our "silent partners for good health" (Huffnagle 2007).

We are constantly bombarded by bad bacteria. Have you ever seen the experiment where you place your hands under UV light and compare them after you have washed them? It's pretty disgusting. We touch so many things in our daily lives. You can actually grow the bacteria you find on your hands in a petri dish and see for yourself what they can turn into. So what is good bacteria, and why does good bacteria matter?

Antibiotics can kill off good bacteria, making a person susceptible to yeast overgrowth, especially when their immune system isn't in peak condition for fighting other invaders. But killing off bad bacteria can also leave the patient susceptible to illness. In clinical trials, mice delivered via C-section and given antibiotics were left immunocompromised. The womb in general is a sterile environment, but once the newborn emerges, the baby is exposed to good and bad microbes. If the baby is delivered vaginally, they are exposed to the microflora in the vagina, which is swallowed. Expecting mothers should want to have the best biome ready for their baby. If a baby is delivered via C-section, they are not exposed to these microbes. If the baby is breastfed, they are exposed to these microbes, but, if not, they are not set up for immune success. Formula doesn't contain the beneficial microbes. There is a lot of existing research comparing the health benefits of being delivered vaginally versus being delivered via C-section, as well as breastfeeding versus using formula, and the results are outstanding (Neu and Rushing 2011). Little ones exposed to a better microbiome have better immune systems, don't get sick as much, have fewer fevers, less diarrhea, and fewer allergies. If a baby is formula fed, it is wise to supplement that child with probiotics, which can help.

The documentary *MicroBirth* discusses how, to an extent, we are all part of a human experiment in that our microbiomes are changing daily.

Our bodies consist of nearly ten trillion cells, and you may be surprised to know that we are also made of over one trillion different microbes, the majority of which live in our intestines. That is why 80 percent of your immune system is in your gut.

Probiotics aren't only beneficial for those little ones growing their microbiome; research exists showing how probiotics can prevent and treat serious chronic diseases in adults, too. Microbes are everywhere. They are in the air we breathe, the ground we walk on, the food we eat—they're even inside us. They make up what we are. Ninety-nine percent of all microbes in our diet are bacteria, while the remaining are yeast or parasites. Our bodies consist of nearly ten trillion cells, and you may be surprised to know that we are also made of over one trillion different microbes, the majority of which live in our intestines. That is why 80 percent of your immune system is in your gut. The rest of the microbes may live in your lungs, on your skin, and in your genital tracts. They are so small that millions can fit into the eye of a needle. There are more of them on a person's hand than there are people on the entire planet.

How do you know if you have more good bacteria than bad? Test. The same stool test I've discussed looks at commensal bacteria, demonstrating the composition, diversity, and relative abundance of gut organisms, all of which are linked to both gastrointestinal and general health. The company I use assesses a key set of twenty-four clinically relevant species.

Easier stated, the stool test I offer to patients can look at which bacteria they are low or high in and if they have yeast or parasites. We can also assess whether the good bacteria that patients are getting from food and probiotic supplements is sufficient. Oftentimes it is not, and patients require much higher doses of probiotics. Two important strains I always assess are the *Lactobacillis* and the *Bifidobacter* species. To simplify, if on a stool test a patient is very low in a *Bifidobacter* species, then we know they need to supplement with it.

Various strains of probiotics can be used to treat various diseases. Probiotics can be used for reasons beyond gastrointestinal health—they can also be used for allergies, eczema, asthma, yeast infections, obesity, and cardiovascular disease. Although we like to think that living in a developed nation means our health should be superior to those in underdeveloped nations, we actually have higher rates of allergies. According to the "hygiene hypothesis," exposure to germs and microbes is actually beneficial to health, as it reduces developing allergies. *The higher the hygiene standards, the cleaner the country, the more allergies.* Isn't that interesting? Probiotics can also help prevent and treat asthma, as they help to reduce inflammation and help to keep the immune system from being triggered by offenders.

Generally speaking, a good, gut-healing dose of probiotics is at least a billion colony-forming units (CFU). I often start patients on twenty billion CFU in our LB product Probiotic Complex. If patients have taken antibiotics and are working to "rebuild their rainforest," I commonly recommend higher dosing, such as a hundred billion CFU of Advanced Probiotic, at least in the short term. In my practice, when patients have diarrhea we use higher dosages. Several studies have shown the benefits of high-dose probiotics in inflammatory bowel disease (IBD), whether Crohn's or colitis, and even in irritable bowel syndrome (Guilliams 2011). For these cases, I use 225 billion CFU in Probiotic Ultra short term, and sometimes I use a prescription product called VSL no. 3 with 450 billion CFU.

An old myth is that probiotics need to be rotated. There is no published evidence supporting this. Also, probiotics for the most part no longer have to be refrigerated. Most companies have moved toward a shelf-stable product, so if the probiotic is taken out of the fridge and left on the shelf it doesn't lose any potency. It's also not a big deal if you miss a dose. The organisms actually last around two weeks in your GI system, so, if you forget a dose, know that organisms you took previously are still in there working for you (Ortho Molecular Products).

Probiotics have a tremendous track record for safety. Toxicity studies in animals have never shown any adverse events or bacteremia (bacteria in the blood) as a result of taking probiotics. In 1999, a large review study examining probiotic use reported no adverse events in 143 clinical trials (Klaire Labs 2012).

The intestinal tract harbors over an estimated hundred trillion microorganisms, but there are currently no "upper safe limits" when dosing probiotics. Some studies have demonstrated effectiveness in the trillions (ibid). One can intuitively assess the safe level of intake of probiotics. Infants and children will take less, while adults are dosed higher. *The only individuals who should not take probiotics are those who are severely immunocompromised.*

In the reinoculation phase, not only do I recommend patients add good bacteria like probiotics, but I also recommend **prebiotics**, which we'll discuss more soon. Not all patients benefit from this however, and some even get worse. If you don't tolerate probiotics or prebiotics well, you could have SIBO. Why? Remember, SIBO is caused by too much bacteria, including good bacteria. When I had SIBO, I found that taking probiotics worsened my symptoms. This is for the same reason that some patients with SIBO may not tolerate prebiotics like fiber.

I tell patients to think of prebiotics as food for the good bacteria (probiotics), or as a fiber that acts as a fertilizer for the good bacteria. The top supplement sources of prebiotics that I use are inulin, arabinogalactins, and fructooligosaccharides (FOS). **FOS** are sugars that are linked together in chain formation. **Inulin** is a popular type of FOS; it is a polysaccharide from plants and belongs to the dietary class of fructans. Patients with SIBO or patients avoiding the FODMAPs mentioned previously tend not to tolerate these well, because FOS and inulin both feed probiotic bacteria and opportunistic bacteria in the gut. **Chicory-derived inulin** is best known for its ability to sustain increases in populations of *Bifidobacterium* and *Lactobacillus*. It escapes digestion and absorption in the small intestine, moving to the large intestine to feed your microbiome there (Klaire Labs 2016). This is helpful in a patient who doesn't have SIBO. **Arabino-**

galactans are polysaccharides from the western larch tree, a highly soluble dietary fiber that also stimulates the *Lactobacillus* species. "Arabinogalactan is metabolized to short-chain fatty acids (acetate, butyrate, and propionate) and reduces ammonia production" (Klaire Labs 2016). You may have heard of **psyllium**, which also can have positive effects on stimulating growth of good bacteria. As you can imagine, the side effects of prebiotics are flatulence, bloating, cramps, abdominal discomfort and pain, and diarrhea. Therefore, they should be introduced slowly.

How do you know if you need these? Again, you can be tested. Within the comprehensive stool analysis is a section called Short-Chain Fatty Acids, a metabolomic indicator of GI microbiome health. These indicate whether the patient needs more fiber or prebiotics in their diet.

PHASE 4: REPAIR

The fourth R in a gut-healing protocol stands for **Repair**.

During the Repair phase, the patient adds nutrients to promote proper repair of the intestinal lining, working to further heal their leaky gut. The focus here is to heal the tight junctions in the gut and to reduce overall inflammation. The top agents I recommend for gut repair and healing are the amino acid L-glutamine, zinc, fish oil, and turmeric.

How do you know if your gut is inflamed? First, assume it is inflamed if you have numerous food sensitivities. However, there is also a test for it—the comprehensive stool test I offer to my patients contains several inflammation markers.

Glutamine

Let's start with gut-healing nutrients like L-glutamine. When you purchase glutamine, look for a product that says "L-glutamine." L-glutamine is the most abundant amino acid in the body, and a main source of fuel for the cells of the small intestine. Enterocytes use the amino acid to help maintain the health of the mucosa. Think of glutamine as enhancing the intestine's protective mucosal lining. Even the US Army Medical Research Institute has studied glutamine as an important nutrient to improve gut barrier function (Wilmore 1999). It is also essential for tissue repair throughout the body. Many athletes use L-glutamine for muscle repair, because glutamine is important in the preservation of muscle mass. Similarly, it can be used for gut repair.

I've known individuals with ulcers or suspected digestive issues to juice cabbage. Cabbage is nurturing to the gut because it is high in glutamine. Other foods high in glutamine are bone broth, grass-fed beef, nuts, wild-caught seafood like salmon and spirulina.

Another common reason individuals may supplement with glutamine is to help curb cravings for sugar and alcohol. Cooking and heating inactivates glutamine. I recommend that patients use it in a cold smoothie in the morning.

Gut-healing doses are usually at least 3,000 mg or three grams per day. Many functional medicine providers use higher doses of six to nine grams per day in the short term. Remember, glutamine makes a leaky gut less leaky. It also helps to boost hormone growth and helps the brain get rid of toxic ammonia. Patients who have sensitivity to monosodium glutamate (MSG) should take this with caution, as they may convert glutamine into an excitatory glutamate. Do not take this if you have a history of seizures. I don't tolerate glutamine well, as it makes me feel anxious. Taking magnesium with it should reduce these effects.

Zinc citrate

Zinc is an essential mineral widely recognized for its role in gut and immune health. It is a necessary cofactor for hundreds of enzymes. Zinc has been shown to strengthen one's GI barrier function by supporting the structure of tight junctions. Many individuals take zinc when they are sick, as it can help boost immunity. Similarly, it can help heal the gut. It has been found to help patients with Crohn's disease decrease ulcerations.

Fish oil

Depending on where you live, your diet may not be high in fish. I live in Iowa, and I definitely don't have excellent year-round access to fresh wild-caught salmon. You may have heard of the benefits of oily fish like salmon, sardines, and anchovies. A study of overweight Eskimos who ate oily whale blubber—whom you might suspect were at higher risk for cardiovascular disease—actually found that they were at a reduced risk because of the benefits of the oily fish they consumed. The study found that they had higher blood levels of omega-3s (Dyerberg, Hand, and Hjorne 1975).

Having low levels of omega-3s and higher levels of omega-6s in the diet can lead to increased cardiovascular risk and chronic inflammation. Unfortunately, we are exposed to omega-6s everywhere. Again, living in Iowa, where much corn is grown, high-fructose corn syrup is a big moneymaker here. Corn increases your omega-6s, which then creates a greater need for more omega-3s. Don't get your 3s and 6s confused with your omega-9s. Olive oil is the more common source of omega-9s, but these aren't as anti-inflammatory as omega-3s. High doses of omega-3s, specifically EPA/DHA, have been used in inflammatory bowel diseases like Crohn's and colitis to help reduce the need for steroids as well as reduce inflammatory markers like CRP and sedimentation rate. The average dose I recommend to my patients to reduce inflammation is 3,000 mg of omega-3s, with eicosapentanoic acid (EPA) and docosahexanoic acid (DHA) combined. I advocate for fish oil, specifically. Krill oil isn't as high in EPA/DHA, and a three-gram dose of cod liver contains near toxic levels of vitamin A, unlike fish oil. Even the American Heart Association recommends consumption of EPA/DHA daily.

Turmeric (curcumin)

Gut healing also involves taking natural anti-inflammatories like turmeric. Turmeric—a root in the same family as ginger—has been used for centuries in other cultures as a spice and coloring agent, as well as for its medicinal properties. An extract of turmeric (called curcumin), like ibuprofen, inhibits COX and LOX enzymes, without the side effects. Curcumin has also been shown to reduce inflammatory markers in patients with inflammatory bowel syndromes and ulcers. Remember drugs like NSAIDs can contribute to leaky gut. I have realized that my long history of ibuprofen use for menstrual cramps definitely predisposed me to leaky gut. A better gut healing option for reducing pain and inflammation is to substitute turmeric for ibuprofen. It has an incredible safety record as a powerful anti-inflammatory. I recommend doses of 1,000–2,000 mg/day. LB Turmeric Support is one capsule option.

> **Two of my favorite combination LB powder products for helping patients heal their guts are called Gut Shield and GI Support.**

Gut Shield contains glutamine and zinc as well as a few other key ingredients. **N-acetyl-D-glucosamine** is a mucin precursor that has been shown to increase the production of mucus within the GI tract. This is beneficial in coating the tract and protecting it. Gut Shield also contains **deglycyrrhized licorice root extract (DGL)**, a form of licorice root that doesn't contain glycyrrhizin (which can raise blood pressure) (Deters, Petereit, Schmidgall, and Hensel 2008). Licorice has long been known to treat and heal ulcers. It works as a demulcent to soothe the irritated tissue. It is also anti-spasmodic, anti-inflammatory, and anti-allergenic. **Aloe vera** has been used throughout history to promote a normal inflammatory response. You may have used it on your cuts, scrapes, or burns. Studies have shown that aloe vera is also specifically beneficial to the gastric mucosa, in part through its ability to balance stomach acid levels and promote healthy mucus production (Yusuf, Agunub, and Diana 2004).

All these gut-healing nutrients are packed into one little scoop of powder that can be added to a beverage of your choice or mixed into a smoothie. I recommend patients consume this consistently for at least three months.

My second favorite product for gut healing is called GI Support, a gut-healing protein powder containing glutamine. GI Support is loaded with natural anti-inflammatories such as turmeric. It also contains arabinogalactins, which I discussed in the section on phase 3, Reinoculate. Additionally, GI Support contains **green tea extract (EGCg)**, a potent antioxidant that further helps to reduce inflammation.

Patients commonly ask me how to eat to heal their gut after having removed their food sensitivities. I suggest they memorize the recipe for bone broth, which our ancestors made using essentially the leftover parts of animals they hunted. When you let bones sit on the stove or in a crock pot long enough, they release into the water amino acids like glutamine, proline, and glycine, in addition to collagen. Proline is necessary for collagen production, which strengthens hair, skin, and nails. Glycine is helpful for detoxification, and is also a calming neurotransmitter that helps sleep and memory. Cooking bone broth also releases minerals, which I will discuss in the next chapter. Minerals activate enzymatic processes required for our body to function well.

Gut-Healing Bone Broth

Purchase animal bones or use left overs from meat you have cooked. Chicken bones can cook for 24+ hours, beef bones for 48+ hours, and fish bones for 24+ hours. Avoid bones from GMO fed, antibiotics given animals. Use bones from pasture raised animals and wild-caught fish. Best if used or frozen within a week.

DIRECTIONS

1. Add 1-1.5 pounds bones into a large 8 quart pot and fill with water allowing for boiling room
2. Add 2 tbsp apple cider vinegar to water prior to boiling
3. Consider adding 1 stalk celery, 1 small peeled, chopped onion, 3 chopped carrots
4. Add 1.5 tsp sea salt
5. Heat water slowly, bring to a boil, then allow to simmer for >6 hours time
6. Remove scum if it appears
7. When you are ready, strain the broth, waste the bones
8. Pour into glass containers for storage

INGREDIENTS

- 1-1.5 pounds bones
- 2 tbsp apple cider
- 1 stalk celery
- 1 small onion
- 3 carrots
- 1.5 tsp sea salt

I find it easier to use a scoop of Ancient Nutrition's Bone Broth Protein powder, containing twenty grams of protein. This product also comes in a variety of delicious flavors that you can even cook with. It is an easy way to add protein to muffins, pancakes, and other treats.

PHASE 5: REBALANCE

The fifth R stands for **Rebalance**. There's no pill or diet change you can make to truly remove lifestyle stressors. If your lifestyle is full of stress, this can affect your foundation—your gut health. It's important to take the time to exercise, consider yoga and meditation for stress reduction, and optimize your sleep.

Summary

Remember that food sensitivities and gut infections can contribute to leaky gut and cause a slew of symptoms. To have a healthy "foundation," you must remove the identified foods and treat the identified infections. Just as your home's concrete foundation must have strong footings, your body's foundation may be more likely to suffer from cracks and erosion without addressing all of the five Rs.

To build and maintain a healthy, strong GI foundation, you must **Remove**, **Replace**, **Reestablish**, **Repair**, and **Rebalance**. You must remove your food sensitivities and GI infections to fix the GI permeability, reduce inflammation, and optimize your digestion and absorption of nutrients.

After my patients have followed this process, we discuss weaning off proton pump inhibitors (reflux medications). Many patients were never tested to determine the root cause of the problem before being put on these medications the day they first went to their primary care provider's office. It often takes months to see a gastrointestinal specialist, and by that time these patients have been blocking necessary acid production, which helps kill certain bacteria—potentially inhibiting killing the infection that could've been the initial cause of the reflux—ultimately worsening their undetected gastrointestinal infections. We must work on all the steps mentioned in this chapter to heal the gut, and then, hopefully, wean the patient off their medications.

When the patient is suffering from a leaky gut situation, malabsorption of nutrients can occur. In these instances, I often recommend another comprehensive test, a nutritional evaluation—the topic of chapter 4.

Remember Jennifer, from the beginning of this chapter? She is now migraine-free. She is still dealing with the results of her chronic inflammation, but she remains thankful that the cause of her inflammation was found when it was. Her foundation was not strong; her gut was a mess. She is now sharing her journey with her family, and in doing so she found that her teenage nephew was struggling because he also had so many nutritional deficiencies. He was tested for food sensitivities and celiac and, after changing his diet and lifestyle, is now thriving.

I have been gluten-free for years now. If I can resolve my SIBO and fix my digestion, so can you.

Longevity Blueprint 5-R Nutraceutical Products

Here are my favorite Longevity Blueprint gut-healing products:

1. REMOVE

- Advanced Yeast Complex
- Pylori Essentials

2. REPLACE

- HCL & Pepsin
- Enzyme Support
- Digestive Support (HCL, bile, and enzymes)

3. REINOCULATE

- Probiotic Complex (20 billion CFUs)
- Advanced Probiotic (100 billion CFUs)
- Probiotic Ultra (225 billion CFUs)
- Beneficial Yeast

4. REPAIR

- Gut Shield
- GI Support
- DGL
- Turmeric Support
- Omega-3s

Gluten, dairy, egg-free protein powder options:

- organic hydrobeef
- pea
- rice
- hemp
- collagen

To learn more about the products here as well as the testing companies we use, visit **www.yourlongevityblueprint.com**.

Chapter 1 Resources

FODMAP Friendly: http://fodmapfriendly.com

Home science tools: www.hometrainingtools.com/a/bacteria-handwashing-newsletter

Klaire Labs: www.klaire.com/techarticles.htm

SIBO—small intestine bacterial overgrowth: www.siboinfo.com

Ortho Molecular Products: www.orthomolecularproducts.com

Quest Diagnostics test center: www.questdiagnostics.com

SCD Lifestyle: http://scdlifestyle.com/2012/03/how-to-supplement-with-betaine-hcl-for-low-stomach-acid

Chapter 1 References

1. Blum, Susan. *The Immune System Recovery Plan.* New York: Scribner, 2013.
2. Bohager, Tom. *Everything You Need to Know About Enzymes.* Austin, Texas: Greenleaf Book Group Press, 2009.
3. Campbell-McBride, Natasha. *The Gut and Psychology Syndrome.* Cambridge, England: Medinform Publishing, 2010.
4. Mayo Clinic. "Celiac disease." Mayo Foundation for Medical Education and Research (July 29, 2017). http://www.mayoclinic.org/diseases-conditions/celiac-disease/home/ovc-20214625.
5. Champagne, E.T. "Low gastric hydrochloric acid secretion and mineral bioavailability." *Advances in Experimental Medicine and Biology* 249. (1989):173–84. https://www.ncbi.nlm.nih.gov/pubmed/2543192.
6. Bulletproof Inc. "Coconut Charcoal Capsules Instructions." bulletproof.com (Accessed 2017). http://www.bulletproof.com/coconut-charcoal-capsules-90-ct.
7. Crook, William. *The Yeast Connection Handbook.* Jackson, Tennessee: Professional Books, 2007.
8. Davis, William. *Wheat Belly.* London, England: Harper Thorsons, 2011.

9. Deters, Alexandra, Frank Petereit, Jörg Schmidgall and Andreas Hensel. "N-Acetyl-D-glucosamine oligosaccharides induce mucin secretion from colonic tissue and induce differentiation of human keratinocytes." Journal of Pharmacy and Pharmacology 60. 2008. 197-204.

10. Dyerberg, J., Bang, H.O., and Hjorne, N. (1975). "Fatty acid composition of the plasma lipids in Greenland Eskimos," *American Journal of Clinical Nutrition* 9, no. 28 (1975): 958–66. https://www.ncbi.nlm.nih.gov/pubmed/1163480

11. Fedewa, Amy, and Satish, S.C. "Dietary fructose intolerance, fructan intolerance and FODMAPs." Current *Gastroenterology Reports* 1, no. 16 (January 2014). https://www.ncbi.nlm.nih.gov/pmc/articles/PMC3934501/.

12. Food Allergy Research and Education. "Food allergy facts and statistics for the U.S." foodallergy.org (accessed August 21, 2017). https://www.foodallergy.org/file/facts-stats.pdf.

13. Juntti, H., S. Tikkanen, J. Kokkonen, O.P. Alho, and A. Niinimäki. "Cow's milk allergy is associated with recurrent otitis media during childhood." *Acta Oto-Laryngologica* 8, no. 199 (1999): 867-73.

14. Mayo Clinic. "Fructose intolerance: Which foods to avoid?" Mayo Foundation for Medical Education and Research (Accessed August 22, 2017). http://www.mayoclinic.org/fructose-intolerance/expert-answers/faq-20058097.

15. Gaby, A. *Nutritional Medicine.* Concord, New Hampshire: Fritz Perlberg Publishing, 2011.

16. Gates, Donna. *The Body Ecology Diet.* Hazelwood, Missouri: Hay House, 2011.

17. Guilliams, Thomas. "An Emerging Trend of High Dose Probiotic Use in Clinical Practice," *The Point Institute*, October 2011.

18. Gujral, Niyana, Hugh Freeman, and Alan Thomson. "Celiac disease: Prevalence, diagnosis, pathogenesis and treatment." *World Journal of*

Gastroenterology 42, no. 18 (2012). https://www.ncbi.nlm.nih.gov/pmc/articles/PMC3496881.

19. Hadjivassiliou, Marios, David Sanders, Richard Grünewald, Nicola Woodroofe, Sabrina Boscolo, and Daniel Aeschlimann. "Gluten sensitivity: From gut to brain." *Lancet* 3, no. 9 (2010). http://www.thelancet.com/journals/laneur/article/PIIS1474-4422(09)70290-X/abstract.

20. Huffnagle, G. *The Probiotics Revolution: The Definitive Guide to Safe, Natural Health Solutions*. New York: Bantam Dell, 2007.

21. Jackson, Jessica R., William Eaton, Nicola Casscella, Alessio Fasano, Deanna Kelly. "Neurologic and psychiatric manifestations of celiac disease and gluten sensitivity." *Psychiatric Quarterly* 1, no. 83 (2012): 91-102. https://www.ncbi.nlm.nih.gov/pmc/articles/PMC3641836/.

22. Klaire Labs, "Probiotics: An extraordinary record of safety." Klaire Labs, Probiotic Safety Update, Summer 2012. http://www.klaire.com/images/Probiotic_Safety_Update_Summer_2012.pdf

23. Lord, Richard S. and J. Alexander Bralley. *Laboratory Evaluations for Integrative and Functional Medicine* ed. 2. Metametrix Institute, 2008.

24. Mayo Clinic. "C. difficile infection." mayoclinic.org (2016). https://www.mayoclinic.org/diseases-conditions/c-difficile/diagnosis-treatment/drc-20351697.

25. Myers, Amy. "Everything you need to know about histamine intolerance." mindbodygreen. (October 3, 2013). https://www.mindbodygreen.com/0-11175/everything-you-need-to-know-about-histamine-intolerance.html.

26. Neu, Joesf and Jona Rushing. "Cesarean versus Vaginal Delivery: Long term infant outcomes and the Hygiene Hypothesis," *Clinics in Perinatology* 2, June 2011, https://www.ncbi.nlm.nih.gov/pmc/articles/PMC3110651/.

27. Ortho Molecular Products. "The Right Probiotic Makes All the Difference." orthomolecularproducts.com.

28. Perlmutter, David, and Kristin Loberg. *Grain Brain*. New York: Little, Brown and Co, 2013.

29. Preston F.E., F.R. Rosendaal, I.D. Walker, E. Briët, E. Berntorp, J. Conard, J. Fontcuberta, M. Makris, G. Mariani, W. Noteboom, I. Pabinger, C. Legnani, I. Scharrer, S. Schulman, F.J. van der Meer. "Increased fetal loss in women with heritable thrombophilia," *Lancet* 9032, 348:913–6 (October 5, 1996). https://www.ncbi.nlm.nih.gov/pubmed/8843809.

30. Quest Diagnostics. "IgA, Serum." (2013). http://www.questdiagnostics.com/testcenter/testguide.action?dc=TH_IgA_Serum.

31. Sahley, Billie, and Katherine Birkner, *Heal with Amino Acids and Nutrients*. San Antonio, Texas: Pain & Stress Publishers, 2011.

32. Sullum, Jacob. "Research Shows Cocaine And Heroin Are Less Addictive Than Oreos," *Forbes*, October 2016, https://www.forbes.com/sites/jacobsullum/2013/10/16/research-shows-cocaine-and-heroin-are-less-addictive-than-oreos/.

33. Teitelbaum, Jacob (2007). *From Fatigued to Fantastic*. New York: Penguin Group, 2007

34. University of Nebraska-Lincoln Institute of Agriculture and Natural Resources. "Prevalence of food allergies." farrp.unl.edu (2017). https://farrp.unl.edu/resources/gi-fas/prevalence-of-food-allergies.

35. Wahls, T. *The Wahls Protocol: A Radical New Way to Treat All Chronic Autoimmune Conditions Using Paleo Principles.* New York: Avery, 2014.

36. Walsh, S.J., and Rau L.M. "Autoimmune diseases: a leading cause of death among young and middle-aged women in the United States," *AMJ Public Health* 9 (September 2000), https://www.ncbi.nlm.nih.gov/pubmed/10983209

37. Wilmore, Douglas. "Military strategies for sustainment of nutrition and immune function in the field." Institute of Medicine (US), Committee on Military Nutrition Research (1999). Washington, D.C.: National Academies Press.

38. Wilson, Lawerence. "How Digestion Works." L.D. Wilson Consultants, Inc. (July 2016). http://drlwilson.com/articles/DIGESTION.htm.https://www.ncbi.nlm.nih.gov/books/NBK230973/.

39. Yusuf, Sadiq, Abdulkarim Agunub, and Mshelia Diana. "The effect of Aloe vera A. Berger (Liliaceae) on gastric acid secretion and acute gastric mucosal injury in rats." *Journal of Ethnopharmacology* 93, (2004): 33–37.

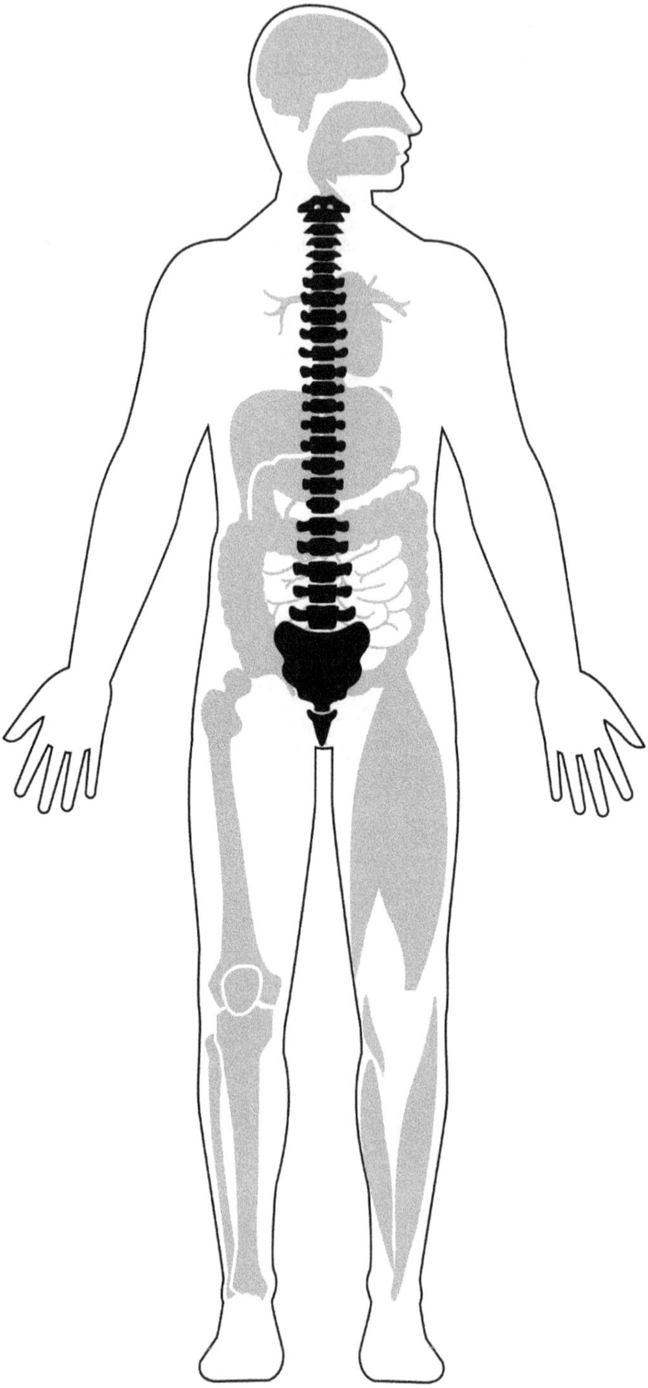

CHAPTER 2

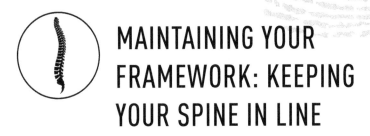

MAINTAINING YOUR FRAMEWORK: KEEPING YOUR SPINE IN LINE

"Medicine is the study of disease and what causes man to die. Chiropractic is the study of health and what causes man to live."

—B.J. Palmer

The frame of a house can never be started until the foundation is complete and level. It's the same with your body. As mentioned in chapter 1, your gut is the foundation of your body, and must be healthy before you move to future steps within the Longevity Blueprint I'm presenting in this book. I cannot emphasize this enough. When building a house, inspectors are brought in with every step in the process to assure the first step was done correctly before the builder can move to the next step.

Contractors need the foundation to be cured and solid. This has to happen before they can build on top of it. Think about it: when a house doesn't settle well, if the foundation isn't solid, it develops cracks in the walls and wavy floors. Similarly, our bodies can become misaligned and develop chronic disease if we don't have both a strong foundation and framework.

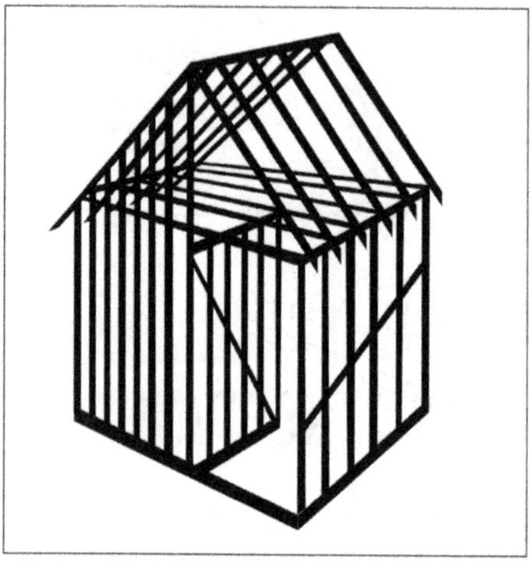

Depending on the weather, for the foundation to settle and become solid, it can take time, even a few weeks. The same is true with your health. You must spend time working to heal your gut, eating clean, removing gut infections, and improving digestion before proceeding to the next step in your Longevity Blueprint.

We all know that a house cannot stand without its supporting structure. Similarly, our bodies can't stand without our musculoskeletal and nervous systems. Our bones are the framework. Just as the framework of the house serves to protect everything inside it (like the plumbing and electrical work), our musculoskeletal system protects our internal organs, like the heart, liver, lungs, stomach, nerves, and more. Our vertebrae protect our spinal cord, and our skull protects our brain.

The framework of a home is slightly flexible. Have you ever been in a high-rise building and felt it moving with the wind? The architect allowed for that give. The same holds true for the spine. The spine is made of several vertebra, which can tolerate some give and take. Typically, a mild curvature of the spine doesn't cause major problems. However, this curvature should be corrected for optimal function of our bodies. We also all have natural curves that we want to maintain. We want the cervical and lumbar spine to have a slight lordosis (inward curvature), and the thoracic spine to have a slight kyphosis (outward curvature).

I was raised in a family that always went to the chiropractor to assess our body's framework and make sure our spines were restored back to proper alignment, and we really never became sick. Seeing a great chiropractor always came in handy, considering my brothers and I were all trained gymnasts. As with many sports, a slight hard landing or a fall off one of the apparatuses could leave me with an acute injury. Even back then when I was very flexible, a slight miscalculation could land me back in the chiropractor's office. Not only did we see the chiropractor for our acute injuries, my parents also taught me from a young age the importance of maintaining my spine with routine adjustments as well.

Your nervous system controls blood flow to organs for them to function, and if the blood flow or nerve impulses are impaired, you can end up with pain or even lowered organ function. Have you ever woken up with a pinched nerve? I have definitely felt that sensation in my upper back and neck upon waking. It's pretty difficult to drive when you can't turn your neck side to side. Oftentimes, a quick trip to my chiropractor to get that vertebra back into place and to get the muscles/ligaments and tendons supported with soft tissue care solves the problem. Why? As my chiropractor and friend Calla Jayne Kleene, DC, says, "Oftentimes that pain is caused by a nerve trapping or impingement in the vertebra, or even out in the periphery from adhesions in muscles. Once a hypomobile joint is adjusted into position, pressure on the nerve is relieved and that pain can resolve."

The same thing can happen with any bone. Ever been short of breath due to a rib dislocating? I have, and it is not comfortable. I think I've dislocated (or broken) every finger and toe at least once in my life. Chiropractic services are essential to management of those bones and joints, getting them back into place so they can heal appropriately.

Two brothers who once came to my office, Collin, age sixteen, and Conner, age seventeen, were both suffering from headaches. Collin was a classically trained pianist, who by the age of sixteen was phenomenal, and Conner was a die-hard sports fanatic. Collin was a perfectionist, not just with his piano but also with academics. He was the head of his high school's honor society, was active in debate, and took several advanced courses. Yet, his mother was concerned about how seriously he was taking his life. His goal was to obtain a college scholarship, so he had piano recitals nearly once a month, and he often didn't sleep the night before. His brother, Conner, played baseball and basketball year 'round. He wasn't the largest guy on his team, but he was known as the toughest, pushing others around on the court and on the field before they could push him around. Although the brothers' daily routines were very different, they ate similar family meals, and they each had nagging headaches that presented at different times.

NERVOUS SYSTEM

Your **nervous system** is made up of nerve cells (**neurons**). Like all other cells, neurons require oxygen and nutrients to survive. Your nervous system is the part of your body that transmits signals to stop or start processes. It helps you communicate with the world. Your **central nervous system** (CNS) includes the brain and spinal cord.

The brain is the master computer and your spinal cord relays information from the brain. Your **peripheral nervous system** (PNS) is the part of the nervous system that branches outside of the brain and spinal cord. It includes the nerves running through your hands, feet, skin, mouth, and organs, and receives signals from, and sends signals to, the CNS.

The nervous system takes in information through the senses and processes that information. Muscles need innervation to move; you may reflexively pull your hand back from a hot burner—the nervous system controls those movements.

The **somatic nervous system** (*voluntary* nervous system) controls everything that we are conscious of, and can choose to influence that consciousness—for instance, moving our arms to pick up a book, or typing this page, or moving our legs to walk. The **autonomic nervous system** (*involuntary* nervous system) regulates the processes in the body that we cannot consciously control or influence. It's constantly regulating breathing, heartbeat, and metabolic processes. It tells the brain that the bladder is full. It controls body temperature, circulation, and sweat.

The autonomic nervous system is made up of three parts: the sympathetic nervous system, the parasympathetic nervous system, and the enteric (gastrointestinal) nervous system.

The **sympathetic nervous system** triggers the body's *fight-or-flight response*. It helps your heart beat faster and opens your airways to breathe more easily if you're dealing with a fearful situation. It also inhibits digestion at those times, which is especially useful in times of emergency.

The **parasympathetic nervous system** is just the opposite. It helps you rest and digest. It is responsible for the bodily functions when you are at rest, including digestion. It helps you to relax.

The **enteric nervous system** is a separate nervous system for the bowels only, helping to regulate bowel motility and digestion.

Sympathetic nerves arise from the middle of our spinal cord and extend outward, communicating messages out to the body.

Since your nervous system controls and coordinates every single function in your body, you want a properly functioning spine that is ready and able to relay every important piece of information. It's possible now to receive an alert on your smartphone when the temperature of your home drops too high or too low. At your order, the digital command center will then turn on the heat or air for your comfort. What if your spine and nervous system can send the same signals? If you have a headache, tingling, or pain in general, your body is telling you something. You need good, functional spinal motion, free of subluxations (misalignments), with good muscle tone to help keep the nervous system relaying vital information from your stomach to your brain and back. You need that functional motion to keep the information exchange—the highway—open, giving your brain vital information about what is going on 24/7. Anything that damages or stresses your nervous system will affect these signals and have effects on the rest of your body.

How is it determined if you are dead or alive? Not by your heart or lungs, but by the activity of your brain. Did you know that when an egg is fertilized and life begins, the first cells created are the brain and spinal cord? Once nerves are developed, buds form at the ends, which develop into all of our vital organs. Our central nervous system is the beginning of life, and continues to control life. You can't live without your central nervous system—your brain and spinal cord.

NERVOUS SYSTEM

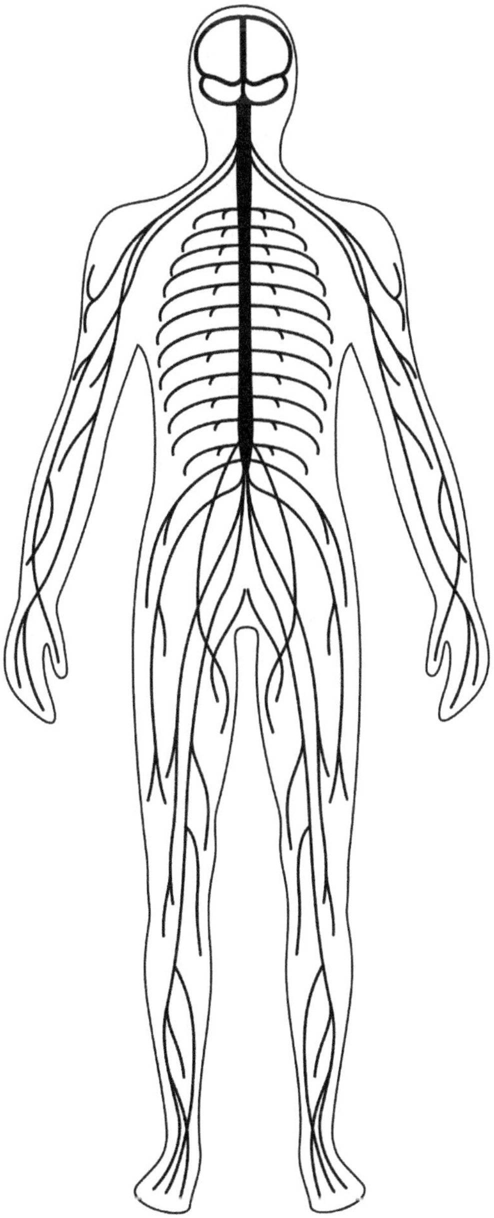

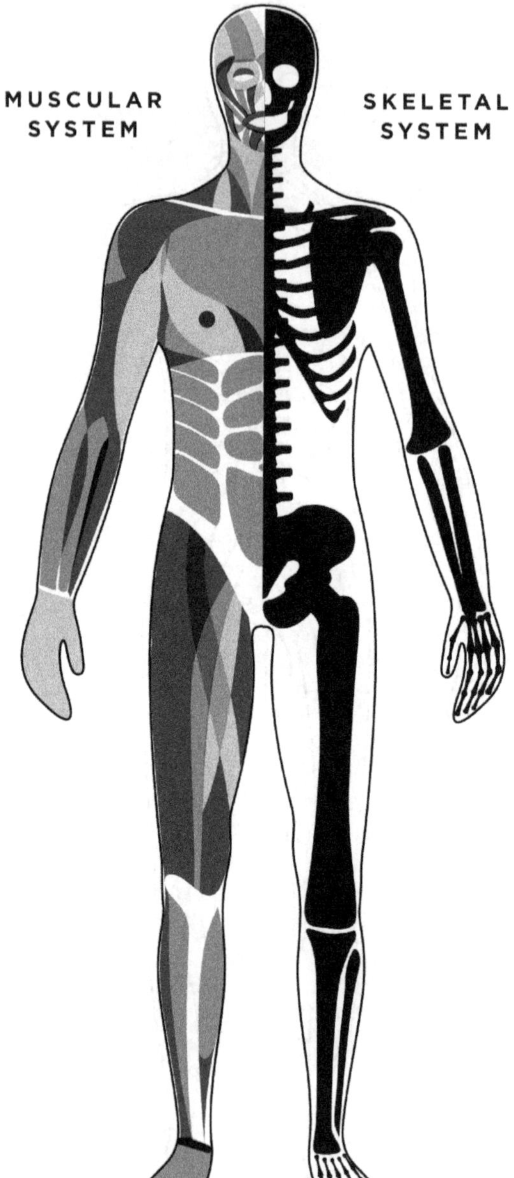
MUSCULAR
SYSTEM
SKELETAL
SYSTEM

MUSCULOSKELETAL SYSTEM

The musculoskeletal system provides us form, support, stability, and mobility. It is made up of the 206 bones of the skeleton, six to eight hundred muscles, cartilage, tendons, ligaments, joints, and other connective tissues that support and bind tissues and organs together. The skull bones protect the brain, the spine protects nerves in the spinal cord, and the ribs protect organs like the lungs, heart, and liver. The bones provide protection and support through movement. The bones and muscles, working in tandem, allow us to function. Bones are held in place by muscles, and are connected by ligaments to form joints to allow for motion. Cartilage prevents our bone ends from rubbing directly against each other in the joints, which can cause pain. The bones, along with muscles and ligaments, provide stability to the spine. While ligaments connect bones to other bones, tendons connect bones to muscles.

Nerves receive information from the brain and are in constant communication with our muscles. The muscles are all under the control of the nervous system, and they help to protect it. The most common bone and joint diseases are osteoporosis and osteoarthritis.

Osteoporosis

Osteoporosis is the most common bone disorder in America, occurring in 50 percent of women, leading to 1.5 million fractures each year (Office of the Surgeon General 2004). Spinal compression fractures may cause a deformed spine, height loss, pain, appetite loss, heartburn, bloating, and difficulty breathing.

You may not realize that your bones are constantly changing. If you gain weight, your bones need to become stronger to support the load. For instance, if you start a couch-to-5K training program, your muscles will create a positive load on your bones, molding them and creating better stability, literally increasing bone density. Our bones start out as **cartilage**. Then **osteoblasts**, which are bone *builders*, help to change cartilage to bone when we are young, and they continue to remodel our bones as we age. They lay the matrix that makes up our bones. This matrix contains collagen, calcium, and phosphates (called hydroxyapatite).

Calcium is important for bones, but it is also important for our muscles and nervous system. If the calcium level in your blood drops too low, your **osteoclasts**, which are bone *breakers*, steal calcium from the bones to meet the needs of other parts of the body.

Healthy bones under a microscope should look like a honeycomb. When an individual has osteoporosis, the holes become larger, and the bone is said to be more porous. As a result, these bones become weaker and are more likely to break. This greatly increases the risk of fractures.

Women who have had a hysterectomy or are postmenopausal are at higher risk for osteoporosis. This is specifically because of the resulting hormone decline. Estrogens keep osteoclasts (bone breakers) at bay. When estrogen is low, osteoclast activity can increase. Steroid and reflux medications can also contribute to bone loss, because they reduce hormone production and nutrient absorption, respectively.

Additional risk factors for osteoporosis include being older, being a woman, having a thin stature, being of Caucasian and Asian ethnicity, not exercising, alcoholism, smoking, crash dieting, eating disorders, and nutritional deficiencies like calcium and Vitamin D.

Osteoporosis is often detected by a dual-energy x-ray absorptiometry (DEXA) scan, also called a bone density scan. A T-score of 0 means your bone mineral density (BMD) is equal to the norm for a healthy young adult. Osteopenia occurs when BMD is between 1 and 2.5 standard deviations below peak young adult BMD (T-score between -1 to -2.5). Osteoporosis occurs when BMD ≥ 2.5 standard deviations below normal (T-score is -2.5 or lower). If you had an unusual fracture unexpectedly at a young age, it is beneficial to have your BMD tested. I've seen women in their twenties and thirties already with osteoporosis, some from low hormone levels if their period cycles have been irregular of stopped. Also, every postmenopausal woman should have a bone density test to assess her baseline to know if she is already osteopenic or osteoporotic. Some believe that fracture risk could be as high as 20 percent for those with osteoporosis. Fractures increase the risk of death. Several studies have shown that an osteoporosis fracture in men or women increases the risk of dying within five to ten years following the injury compared to the normal population (Bluic et al. 2009). To reduce this risk, those with bone density issues should be treated.

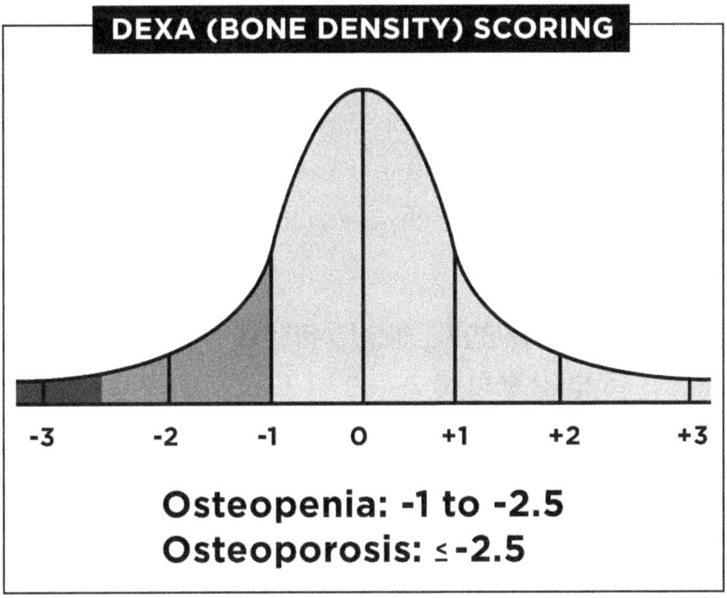

Osteoarthritis

Osteoarthritis (OA) is also known as degenerative joint disease. It can progress slowly, often starting as morning stiffness. It is the most common chronic condition of the joints, and affects twenty-seven million individuals every year (Arthritis Foundation). It is the leading cause of disability in the United States. OA can affect any joint, but most commonly affects the knees, hips, lower back, and neck. A normal joint contains a rubbery material called **cartilage** that covers each end of the bone. This cartilage acts as a cushion, and is made up of collagen and chondroitin sulfate. It allows for the smooth, gliding movement in the joint, reducing pressure. When this cartilage wears down, the cushion is gone and pain can occur. The cartilage can wear away to the point where bone rubs on bone, leading to worsening joint damage and more pain.

Much back pain is due to degenerative disc disease in the spine, another term for osteoarthritis. Like other joints in the body, each vertebral segment is a joint that has cartilage in it. In between the vertebral body and each disc is a layer of cartilage, and when this starts to wear down, inflammation can set in. Inflammation is often the cause of the disc narrowing as well. You want your discs well nurtured so that they don't dehydrate and collapse.

TESTING OPTIONS FOR BONE, JOINT, MUSCLE, AND NERVE (BRAIN) HEALTH

Clinicians who are skilled in assessing musculoskeletal injuries can often deduce based on a physical exam what injury has taken place. Physical therapists are experts in assessing problematic areas. They help patients improve or restore mobility and can help reduce pain. They are experts at helping patients improve strength and stability. Personal trainers can also help patients gain confidence and strength.

However, various testing options exist to confirm those suspicions. During an **x-ray**, beams are passed through your body. Dense materials, such as bone and metal, show up as white on x-rays. The air in your lungs shows up as black. Fat and muscle appear as shades of gray. X-rays can help to detect pneumonia or collapsed lungs, enlargement in your heart, calcium deposits, and fractures. They can also help show broken bones and arthritic joints. A **dual energy x-ray absorptiometry** (DEXA) scan, as I mentioned, is an enhanced form of X-ray technology that measures bone loss.

Magnetic resonance imaging (MRI) uses a magnetic field and radio waves to create detailed images of the organs and tissues within your body. The MRI can produce 3-D images that your provider can view from many different angles. MRIs help identify soft tissue (muscle) injuries. They can help to diagnose aneurysms, spinal cord injuries, strokes, tumors, and even multiple sclerosis. One type of MRI, called a **functional MRI**, can be used to assess damage from a head injury or from disorders such as Alzheimer's disease. A **NeuroQuant** is an even fancier way to analyze brain volumes through MRI. This sophisticated program can also help differentiate biotoxin illnesses (discussed further in chapter 8) by looking at the volume changes—for example, Lyme patients typically have putamen atrophy, and mold patients typically have caudate atrophy.

In regard to testing brain health, I mentioned in chapter 1 the association between gut health and nervous system health is the "gut-brain connection." Interestingly, the majority of our neurotransmitters are made in our gut. Other neurotransmitters are made by the adrenal glands, and others by the brain. **Urine neurotransmitter testing** is controversial, but can be used in combination with other tests to help deduce what neurotransmitters the patient has too much of or needs more of.

Chiropractic care

Chiropractors are health care professionals who diagnose and treat neuromuscular disorders. They manually adjust, or manipulate, the spine. Chiropractors strongly believe that proper alignment of the spine is necessary for optimal functioning of the nervous system. Since the nervous system controls all other systems in your body, any compromise to the spine can lead to other problems within the body.

Palmer College of Chiropractic in Iowa was founded by Daniel David (D.D.) Palmer, who wrote, "Chiropractic embraces the science of life, the knowledge of how organisms act in health and disease, also the art of adjusting the neuroskeleton" (Palmer 2010). He states that the neuroskeleton is the ultimate protector of the central nervous system, and that "when any portion is displaced, it is a disturber of vibration, heat, and other functions" (Palmer 2010). I'm not a chiropractor, but I've been visiting them my entire life. The basic belief behind the practice of chiropractic is that if your spinal vertebrae have lost normal range of motion, there may be a loss of normal function in the muscles and organs associated with those segments. That can then result in a dramatic decrease in sensory feedback to the nervous system, which can then result in an increased stress response in that region of the body.

Within the chiropractic realm, a slight misalignment of the vertebrae is often called a subluxation. This can lead to tight muscles, resulting in lack of proper blood flow to areas where oxygen is needed. Nerves can be impinged, and thus a cascade of negative health consequences can occur. This can manifest in different ways—as constipation, headaches, or carpal tunnel syndrome for one patient, or back pain for another.

Many individuals will seek out chiropractic care for these subluxations if they experience uncomfortable sensations like numbness, tingling, or pain associated with increased pressure or irritation to a nerve, often called a pinched nerve.

Chiropractors work to find these subluxations in order to remove any barriers to normal joint and muscle function, and can identify them even before we experience pain. Just as you maintain your car, scheduling your tires' rotation and balance, your body also benefits from regular maintenance. Personally, when I seek chiropractic treatment, I feel more balanced and less stressed, especially with maintenance every month.

Palmer opened his office of magnetic healing in Davenport, Iowa, and gave the first chiropractic adjustment in 1895. He first identified the three causes of vertebral subluxations, which he describes as the Three Ts—thoughts, trauma, and toxins. We live in a society that values a quick fix, and chiropractic can often provide that, but there are times that it can't. I've heard of patients seeing chiropractors for a headache and the headache resolves after one session, while others commit to fifty treatments over two years and their headaches never improve. Keep in mind that the root cause of the subluxation can be different for each patient, and that if the patient and provider never work to correct the thoughts, trauma, or toxins, a simple chiropractic manipulation won't solve the problem.

In addition to chiropractic, there are a number of ways to improve bone, joint, muscle, and brain health:

TIPS FOR BONE, JOINT, AND MUSCLE HEALTH

- Regular chiropractic care
- Positive thinking
- Posture improvement
- Daily stretching
- Healthy eating
- Regular weight-bearing exercise
- Optimize your hormones

Negative thinking, along with the tight muscles and the stressed state that accompanies it, can lead to subluxations. The first thing you can do to prevent these subluxations is to reduce your stress, change your mindset, and limit your toxic burden (more on this in chapter 5). Several books have been written on the benefits of positive thinking. Reading positive affirmations, getting your mindset right every day, and incorporating other stress-reduction techniques, such as stretching, yoga, and exercise, can be very effective. Yoga has been proven to reduce pain and stress related anxieties (Woodyard 2011).

Ensuring correct posture is also very important. Do you find yourself slouching after lunch? Sitting up straight will help keep the spine in line. Simple stretching may also have more health benefits than you realize. Stress causes your muscles to contract, while stretching helps to loosen them up, helping you relax. Stretching also helps with the release of endorphins, making you feel happier, and can also help to improve flexibility and range of motion, as well as improve blood flow to all your organ systems, not just your muscles. It can also help reduce post-workout soreness.

The trauma of being born—the use of vacuum and forceps, caesarean deliveries, and the use of drugs like Pitocin—can affect our nervous system, and thus our posture, from the beginning. Wearing a heavy backpack through school, texting- and smartphone-crazed postures, wearing heels, and even crossing your legs daily can lead to subluxations.

Chapter 5 of this book is entirely dedicated to toxins, which also can cause inflammation, leading to more subluxations.

Additionally, aside from preventing subluxations, "diet and lifestyle factors, as well as numerous specific natural agents, have tremendous impacts on preserving bone mass, preventing fractures, and even building bone mass" (Guilliams 2004). Reducing consumption of caffeine and soft drinks can also help prevent subluxations. Caffeine and soft drinks are natural diuretics that rob your body of essential bone-building nutrients. Additionally, carbonated beverages will leach minerals from your bones. Studies have shown that increased carbonated soft drink consumption by young girls reduces bone mass density (BMD) and dramatically increases fracture risk (Sámano et al. 2013). And, as I discuss further in chapter 4, drugs also induce micronutrient deficiencies.

My chiropractor offers dry needling in her office, which I've found to be extremely helpful; many physical therapists offer this technique as well. Dry needling is a treatment that involves pushing a very thin needle through your skin and into superficial muscle layers at a specific trigger point. The intent is to help release tight muscle bands, releasing tension in order to improve range of motion and alleviate pain.

Dry needling is different than acupuncture, which can also be helpful for some patients. The intent of acupuncture is to unblock energy meridians, called Qi, creating better balance and flow of energy within the body. Acupuncturists assess lack of Qi through an extensive health history that includes bowel and fecal consistency, frequency, and texture, looking at your tongue, and reading your pulses. They then use needles and herbs to restore Qi energy flow. Acupuncture is a healing art that is vastly misunderstood.

Acupuncture, along with chiropractic—the world of complementary and alternative medicine (CAM)—can be difficult to "prove" effective. It's difficult to eliminate other variables that impact a patient's response to care and treatment in order to prove the treatment is effective, even when medication is involved. To deliver a "sham" adjustment or a "sham" acupuncture session is more difficult than proscribing a placebo medication to a test group. Just touching a patient can have a dramatic effect, especially in the elderly population. Physical and compassionate touch can be beneficial. Do you know the power of a hug? A smile? Think about a physical touch to a painful and achy body. Bedside manner goes a long way in the healing process. Many of the providers in the CAM arena touch their patients at every encounter compared to their medical counterparts. It is an intimate relationship built on trust.

My chiropractic friend, Dr. Kleene, shared a story with me of a patient who "threw his back out" and visited the emergency room the night before coming to her office. His wife carried him into the office. When Dr. Kleene lifted the man's shirt, he had three black spots in his lumbar paraspinal region (lower back). She asked him if they had run x-rays at the ER, and he said they never even touched him—they diagnosed him with a muscle spasm and gave him NSAIDs and pain relievers. We have an entire health care community that does not physically touch patients, especially in musculoskeletal pain situations. Dr. Kleene sent the patient for x-rays and found that he had three avulsion fractures of the transverse processes (vertebral fractures) in his lumbar spine, an impressive injury that had been largely dismissed the night before. Dr. Kleene didn't know whether the bruises had been present the night before, but the fact that the medical providers never even touched this patient—and to diagnose a muscle spasm—is terrible.

Dr. Kleene also offers an Active Release Technique (ART), as well as the Graston Technique, which the creator describes on their website, grastontechnique.com, as an "evidence-based form of instrument-assisted soft tissue mobilization that enables clinicians to detect and effectively break down scar tissue and fascial restrictions as well as maintain optimal range of motion." This works beautifully in conditions like plantar fasciitis, tennis elbow, and carpal tunnel. Look for a chiropractor, or even a physical therapist, certified in offering this technique if you suffer from one of these conditions.

Establishing a high peak bone mass (PBM) by the age of twenty may be one of the most important factors in maintaining strong bones in your elderly years. Having osteoporosis increases fracture risk, increasing risk of death. The mortality rate after a hip fracture can range from 14 to 58 percent (Studd et al. 1990). PBM is best achieved with regular weight-bearing exercise, such as walking, hiking, jogging, climbing stairs, playing tennis, dancing, and weight lifting, which forces you to work against gravity. Exercise promotes blood flow, which helps with healing injuries and maintaining weight. Maintaining a healthy weight is very important, since being overweight adds additional pressure to your joints and back.

Lastly, optimizing hormones can greatly benefit bone density. Replacing estrogen, progesterone, and testosterone in women—and testosterone in men—will help reduce bone loss, and can even help with cartilage renewal. I've seen both female and male patients in my functional medicine practice with osteoporosis or similar conditions who experience joint pain reduction and BMD improvement using natural hormone replacement therapy. However, testosterone replacement via pellet therapy, discussed later in chapter 6, has shown the most dramatic rise in BMD, as great as 8.3 percent (Studd et al. 1990). I have not seen any drug or lifestyle change improve BMD to this degree.

Recently, I had an osteoporotic woman come to my practice for help with her bone density. I placed her on a variety of bone health nutrients and gave her hormone pellets. Within a year her bone density improved by 3.7 percent. That is phenomenal. In my experience, when patients use oral medications such as bisphosphonates for bone density, their provider is satisfied if bone density doesn't worsen. I was elated when I was able to share with this patient that she no longer had osteoporosis.

Bone Health Nutrients

There are several nutrients that can assist with bone and joint health. Most individuals are aware that our bones are composed of calcium and phosphorus. Yes, we need to consume calcium from our diet or from supplements, but your bones need more than calcium.

Vitamin D is mentioned in many chapters in this book. It helps your body absorb calcium and phosphorus from the food you eat, and it is important for bone remodeling by osteoblasts and osteoclasts.

Without enough **magnesium**, **calcium** can collect in the wrong places in the soft tissues and cause arthritis. Therefore, magnesium is just as important as calcium. Two-thirds of the magnesium in our bodies is located within the bones (Castiglioni 2013). Magnesium is very important for osteoporosis, and "represents a helpful intervention to maintain bone integrity" (Castiglioni 2013). A commonly recommended ratio of magnesium to calcium is 2 to 1, although most women consume less magnesium than that. Magnesium activates enzymes involved in forming new calcium crystals, and helps with calcium absorption, as well as converting vitamin D to its active form. If you've had challenges improving your vitamin D level despite high dosing, it may be because you are low in magnesium.

A much-overlooked nutrient for bone health is **vitamin K**. Low levels of vitamin K2 are directly related to reduced BMD. K2 helps bind calcium into the bone. Vitamin K is a primary cofactor in absorption of calcium into bone. It synergistically works with vitamin D3 to improve calcium absorption. Think of vitamin D as the doorman opening the door for calcium to enter the blood stream. Vitamin K is the usher that takes calcium from the lobby and directs it to its appropriate seat in the bone matrix. We carry vitamin D3 products in both liquid and capsule form, with and without K2.

Strontium is another mineral I use in my functional medicine practice for my patients with osteopenia and osteoporosis. Randomized, double blind, placebo controlled clinical trials show that strontium ranelate at a dose of 1 g/day significantly increases bone mineral density compared to placebos, and reduces the incidence of fractures (Reginster et al. 2002). Strontium has previously demonstrated its effectiveness in several different trials (PREVOS, STRATOS, TROPOS, and SOTO). Strontium stimulates new bone growth by helping bone turnover. How does it work? It promotes osteoblastic activity and reduces osteoclastic activity. Our strontium LB product is called Strontium Chelate.

Another one of our LB products, Bone Support, is a bone-building pack we offer to our patients with bone density issues, containing vitamin D3, calcium, magnesium, K2, strontium, and boron. It is also a multivitamin. As you will learn in chapter 4, amino acid chelates are the best-absorbed forms of minerals; they are primarily what I use in my practice, and are what Bone Support contains. Strontium and calcium compete for binding sites, and thus should be taken at separate times throughout the day. In Bone Support, strontium is taken in the morning, and a calcium blend is taken in the evening.

Compare these nutraceutical options to the most commonly prescribed class of medications for osteoporosis—the bisphosphonates, including Fosamax, Boniva, and Actonel—which prevent the loss of bone mass. These drugs are taken up by your bones and cause the osteoclasts that resorb bone to slow down. They don't help you to build bone. Gastrointestinal adverse effects are the most common reason that patients discontinue these drugs. You must sit upright for thirty to sixty minutes after ingesting. The medication can lead to gastrointestinal bleeding, increase the risk of esophageal cancer, and increase the risk of fracture. It can also cause low calcium levels (Kennel and Drake 2009).

Why is it that dentists ask whether you are on bisphosphonates? Because they need to know how frail your bones may be. Have you ever read the package insert on these drugs? "Side effects include osteonecrosis of the jaw." This is a disease of the bone where bone tissue dies and the bone collapses. Dentists need to know this before they start drilling into your mouth. As with every decision we make, we must weigh the risks versus the benefits.

Your bones are constantly turning over. It has been said that every ten years you develop a new skeleton. That is an exaggeration, but you get my point. As you get older, this remodeling process slows down, and your bones become weaker. If you freeze the process with bisphosphonates, you are not as effectively building new bone. A dry, dead tree branch will break very easily, and the same is true of your bones. I've had several patients who were afraid to take bisphosphonates because they knew someone who experienced adverse events from the medication and wanted safer options.

Joint Health Nutrients

There are also several well-known nutrients that can help with overall joint health. Our joints are made of both collagen peptides and glucosamine chondroitin. I often encourage my patients to consume bone broth loaded with collagen, or to take a collagen peptide product. I enjoy Ancient Nutrition collagen protein powders. They easily mix into many drinks and other recipes. Clinical trials have shown that 1.5 g of **glucosamine** was slower to relieve arthritic pain than Advil, but over time was just as effective (Lopes 1982). **Chondroitin sulfate** is another well-known joint-healthy ingredient.

Studied since the 1980s, it helps draw water into the joint tissues and hydrate them. The dose typically used in clinical trials has been about 1,200 mg daily, given as 400 mg three times a day. Trials combining both glucosamine and chondroitin have shown statistically significant improvement for arthritic pain. Our LB product for joint health is called Joint Support. Many of my patients have also benefitted from taking natural anti-inflammatories like our LB product Turmeric Support—mentioned in chapter 1—which contains turmeric.

Our LB product for joint health is called Joint Support.

If natural options aren't helping, pharmaceutical options like aspirin or NSAIDs can be used. Additionally, some medical providers offer joint injections of hyaluronic acid, or synthetic lubricants like Synvisc. The combination can often delay the need for joint replacement surgery.

Muscle Health Nutrients

Have you ever had a hot lower back, sprained ankle, disc irritation, or bursitis? For soft tissue injuries, I often recommend patients try our Soft Tissue Support, which contains turmeric and proteolytic enzymes to help with recovery and repair. It also contains a handful of synergistic ingredients: the herb Boswellia aids in repair and can help reduce the pain, and the proteolytic enzymes help break down fibrinogen to increase blood flow to the affected area, increasing oxygen and reducing healing time.

Compare this to use of an NSAID like ibuprofen. Most people who treat these symptoms with NSAIDs are unaware that these drugs inhibit glucosamine sulfate. By taking the drug, yes, you are inhibiting pain, but unfortunately you are also inhibiting tissue repair and extending your recovery time. Patients report tremendous reduction in swelling when using our Soft Tissue Support product. This can help expedite the healing process.

Nerve/Brain Health Nutrients

There are many brain health supportive nutrients available. Our brains are full of fat, thus consuming healthy fats like omega-3s benefits our mental health.

Also, keeping the nervous system from experiencing high levels of stress is vital. However, stress is not always avoidable. **Phosphatidyl serine** (PS) is a phospholipid found in high concentrations in our brains. It plays an important role in cellular communication. It's very difficult to obtain PS from foods. I often recommend that patients take 100 mg during times of stress. PS will help modulate the stress response and reduce high cortisol. It can be taken at night to help suppress adrenaline so that the individual can sleep. When used consistently, it can help reset the circadian rhythm to keep cortisol lower at night when sleeping.

L-theanine, an amino acid that is useful for calming an overactive nervous system, helps to induce a relaxed state. It is helpful for sleep, anxiety, and stress. I use L-theanine before public speaking or when I feel wired and know I need to calm down. It is discussed further in chapter 4.

Antioxidants play a crucial role in brain health as well. Many antioxidants are mentioned in chapter 4. Antioxidants include resveratrol, alpha lipoic acid (ALA), CoQ10, NAC, glutathione, and vitamin C. Our LB product Antioxidant Support contains resveratrol and glucoraphanin, the equivalent of a cup and a half of broccoli. We also carry ALA, CoQ10 100, and 300 mg of NAC separately.

CONCLUSION

A house cannot stand without its supporting framework. The same is true with our bodies. Exercise has proven time and time again to provide longevity benefits, not just for our memory, but also for our range of motion and bone density. Having your hormones and nutrient levels assessed and optimized can help with bone, joint, and memory health as well. Chiropractic care also has several benefits. However, I do recognize that finding the right chiropractor can be difficult. As Dr. Kleene often tells her patients, "There are over two hundred techniques and philosophies specific to chiropractic and physical medicine. Getting my patients better in a reasonable timeframe is one of my main responsibilities as a chiropractor. A good, ethical chiropractor will refer to either another chiropractor or provider who is trained in a specific technique if their patient's symptoms and case history warrant it."

See a chiropractor trained in sports medicine if your symptoms warrant that. Their training through the McKenzie Institute is the gold standard in managing lumbar and cervical spine disc disorders. Have your infants and children see a pediatric chiropractor. You can find a specialty chiropractor for what you need if you look. A chiropractor who will see a patient thirty-six times for a headache and not think about what else could be causing the symptoms is no better than a doctor giving Tylenol to reduce a fever—it's not a lack of Tylenol that caused the fever. Don't see a chiropractor who falls into the trap of being the "all-natural" Band-Aid; treatment is really about identifying the cause among D.D. Palmer's triggers: thoughts, trauma, and toxins. However, yes, spinal misalignment can cause headaches, and chiropractors are excellent at removing and reducing that burden for many.

That was the case with Conner, one of the two brothers mentioned at the beginning of this chapter. His headaches were caused by overuse of his muscles and joints in all his year-round sports, so he greatly needed chiropractic adjustments to address his "trauma." However, his brother Collin's headaches were of an entirely different origin. As discussed in chapter 1, food sensitivities are often a huge trigger. Collin was eating grilled cheese sandwiches every single day. That's all he felt he had time for between his academics, debate, and piano practice. He also already had stress-induced headaches as a seventeen-year-old. Helping him remove gluten and dairy and find other healthy stress-reduction techniques set him up for improved sleep and improved his performance skills. Ironically, his mother also needed help. She walked notably slow to each of his appointments. Although she wasn't my patient, I asked her about her problems, and she shared that she had been struggling with plantar fasciitis. I sent her to Dr. Kleene, and her symptoms were greatly improved through the Graston Technique, which does the trick nearly every time. I placed Conner and his mother on our Soft Tissue Support to help reduce inflammation and promote healing. Conner loves the product. As a teenager, he takes it with him everywhere, especially for away games.

Remember, if you are heading into a state of chronic symptoms, look to the steps in this Longevity Blueprint. What else might you be neglecting? Is it your nutrition? Is it your gut health? Have you denatured your intestines with long-term use of NSAIDs to mask your musculoskeletal pain? Swap out your NSAIDs for our Soft Tissue Support and continue on the Longevity Blueprint path.

You can maintain your framework following your Longevity Blueprint. Consider maintenance chiropractic care as well as treatment when issues arise. Safe nutrients exist that can work synergistically to help improve your bone, joint, and muscle health.

Longevity Blueprint Nutraceutical Products

Here are my favorite Longevity Blueprint bone/joint/muscle healing products:

- Vitamin D3 1000
- Vitamin D3 5000
- Vitamin D3 5000 + K2
- Liquid D3
- Liquid D3 + K2
- Calcium + Magnesium Chelates
- Magnesium Chelate
- Strontium Chelate
- Bone Support
- Joint Support
- Antioxidant Support
- Soft Tissue Support
- Turmeric Support

Chapter 2 Resources

Graston Technique: www.grastontechnique.com

Chapter 2 References

1. Arthritis Foundation. "What is osteoarthritis?" Retrieved September 27, 2017. http://www.arthritis.org/about-arthritis/types/osteoarthritis/what-is-osteoarthritis.php.

2. Bluic, D., N.D. Nguyen, V.E. Milch, T.V. Nguyen, J.A. Eisman, and J.R. Center. "Mortality risk associated with low-trauma osteoporotic fracture and subsequent fracture in men and women." *Journal of the American Medical Association* 5, no. 301 (February 4, 2009): 513–21.

3. Castiglioni, Sara, Alessandra Cazzaniga, Walter Albisetti, and Jeanette Maier. "Magnesium and osteoporosis: Current state of knowledge and future research directions." *Nutrients* 8, no. 5 (August 2013): 3022–3033. https://www.ncbi.nlm.nih.gov/pmc/articles/PMC3775240/pdf/nutrients-05-03022.pdf

4. Guilliams, Thomas. "Osteoporosis, protecting and strengthening bones naturally," *The Standard* 2, no. (2004).

5. Kennel, K.A., and M.T. Drake "Adverse effects of bisphosphonates: Implications for osteoporosis management." *Mayo Clinic Proceedings* 7, no. 84 (2009):632–38.

6. Office of the Surgeon General (US). *Bone Health and Osteoporosis: A Report of the Surgeon General.* Office of the Surgeon General (US): Rockville, Maryland, 2004.

7. Palmer, Daniel David. The Chiropractor. Whitefish, Montana: Kessinger Legacy Reprints, 2010.

8. Reginster, J.Y., N. Sarlet, E. Lejeune, L. Leonori. "Prevention of early postmenopausal bone loss by strontium ranelate." *Osteoporosis International* 12, no. 13 (2002): 925–31.

9. Reginster, J.Y., E. Seeman, M.C. De Vernejoul, S. Adami, J. Compston, C. Phenekos, J.P. Devogelaer, M.D. Curiel, A. Sawicki, S. Goemaere, O.H. Sorensen, D. Felsenberg, and P.J. Meunier. "Strontium ranelate reduces the risk of nonvertebral fractures in postmenopausal women with osteoporosis: Treatment of peripheral

osteoporosis (TROPOS) study." *Journal of Clinical Endocrinology Metabolism* 5, no. 90 (May 2005): 2816–22.

10. Sámano R., A.L. Rodríguez Ventura, E.Y. Godínez Martínez, B. Rivera, M. Medina Flores, B. Sánchez, H. Martínez Rojano, and C. Ramirez. "Association of consumption of carbonated beverages and decalcification in woman on reproductive and non-reproductive age of Mexico City." *Nutricion Hospitalaria* 5, no. 28 (October 2013): 1750-6. https://www.ncbi.nlm.nih.gov/pubmed/24160242.

11. Studd, J., M. Savvas, N. Waston, T. Garnett, I. Fogelman, and D. Cooper. "The relationship between plasma estradiol and the increase in bone density in postmenopausal women after treatment with subcutaneous hormone implants." *American Journal of Obstetrics & Gynecology* 5 pt. 1, no. 163 (Novemeber 1990): 1474–9. https://www.ncbi.nlm.nih.gov/pubmed/2240090.

12. Vaz, Antonio Lopez. "Double-blind clinical evaluation of the relative efficacy of ibuprofen and glucosamine sulphate in the management of osteoarthrosis of the knee in out-patients." Current Medical Research and Opinion 8, no. 3 (February 1982): 145-9.

13. Woodyard, Catherine. "Exploring the therapeutic effects of yoga and its ability to increase quality of life." International Journal of Yoga 2, no. 4 (2011): 49-51. https://www.ncbi.nlm.nih.gov/pmc/articles/PMC3193654/.

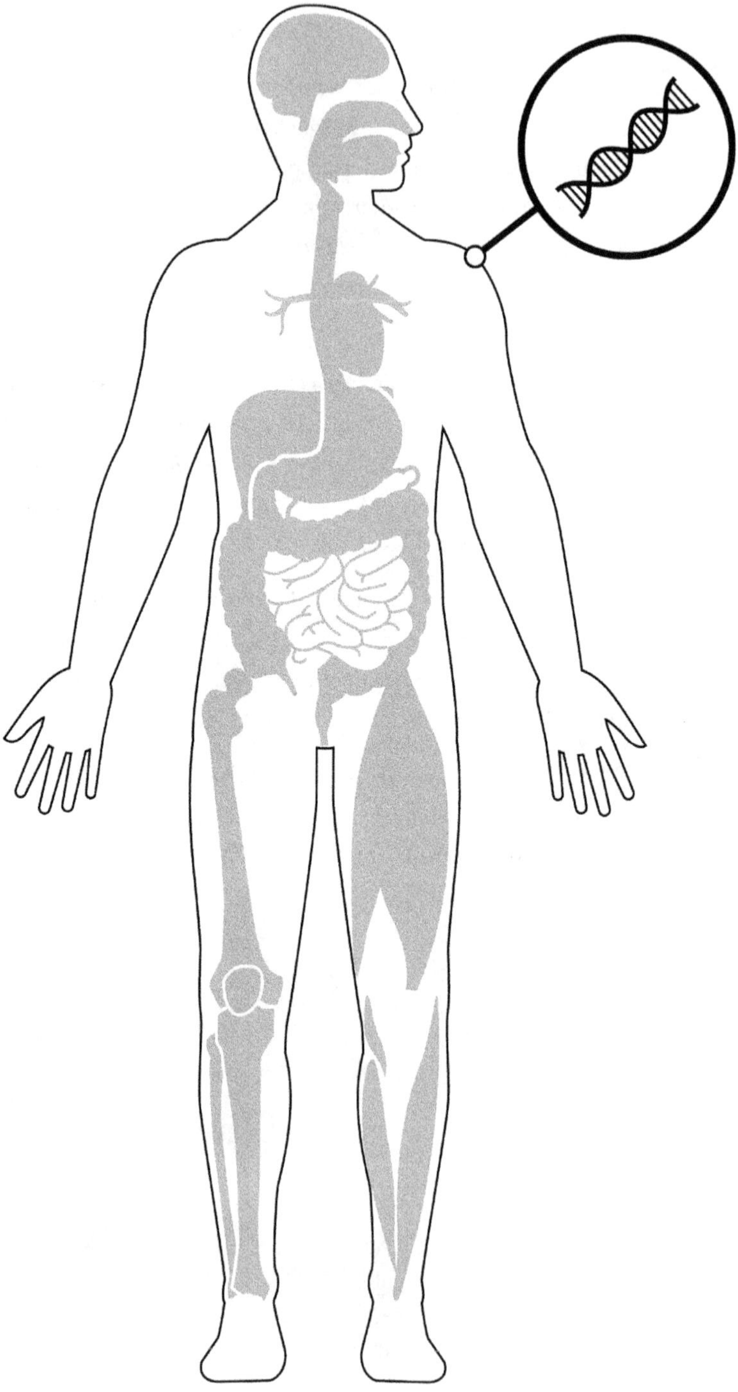

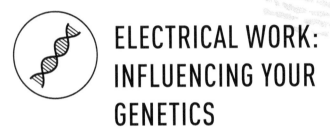

CHAPTER 3

ELECTRICAL WORK: INFLUENCING YOUR GENETICS

Your genetics load the gun. Your lifestyle pulls the trigger.
—Dr. Mehmet Oz

Chelsea was heartbroken and desperate. In her first appointment with me, she shared that she'd had eight miscarriages, most between four and seven weeks gestation. She'd been advised to attempt a very expensive procedure called in vitro fertilization (IVF), and she came to my clinic as a last resort before proceeding. Her period cycles were regular, every twenty-eight days. Home ovulation test strips were nearly always positive around day fourteen. All her hormone levels were normal. She had seen several gynecologists, and none had been able to help her. I had Chelsea undergo the same testing I recommend for most of my patients. Since her first round of testing was normal, I started thinking outside the box. I asked her if she had ever been tested for the methylenetetrahydrofolate reductase (MTHFR) genetic variants; she had not. **Variants** are subtle differences in our DNA. While we were awaiting her results, I told her to stop taking folic acid—which her gynecologist had started her on—as folic acid can actually be dangerous to those with MTHFR variants. Interestingly, her husband had enrolled in a fertility study in which he had also been advised to take folic acid, as well as zinc. I suggested that he also stop taking folic acid, since he too could have MTHFR variants.

We know that environment heavily influences our genes. The saying, "Our genetics load the gun, but environment pulls the trigger" means, in part, that one's environment can be the straw that breaks the camel's back. For instance, you could be managing your genetic variants well at home until you travel. But the factors of traveling—stress, sleep deprivation, radiation and electromagnetic chaos, the mold exposure in the beach house you travel to, combined with the poolside margaritas—can suddenly set off a cascade of events and you'll start to fall apart.

Compare two of my patients with Lyme disease. I've seen one simply require a few months of antibiotics for them to return to normal functioning, while another struggled for decades due to the effects of oxidative stress and inflammation. Why was one path to recovery more difficult? One may have been genetically primed for better success than the other. One may have inherited a "worse" set of genetic variants.

We all have genetic variants. Your goal should be to keep "bad" genes less active and "good" genes working to their full potential. Equating this with the electrical work throughout a house, there's no need to have all the lights turned on at once. When you wake up in the morning, you likely turn on the bedroom and bathroom lights, and then you may turn on the kitchen lights as you prepare breakfast. Have you ever considered the intricate process takes place in the quick second it takes to turn your lights on with the flick of the switch? Similarly, our genes fuel every enzymatic reaction and every cell in our body.

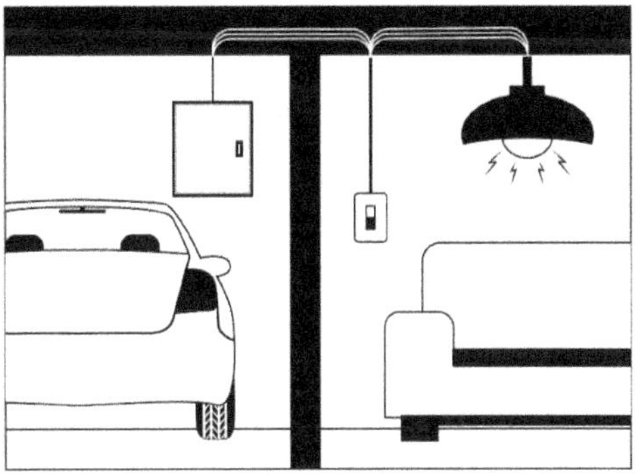

A disrupted supply during power outages and blackouts can stop operations and inconvenience those affected. A power outage is never fun. Also, if you keep a light turned on too long, what happens? It burns out. That is relatively similar to what can happen with genes.

First, some Genetics 101. **DNA** provides the instructions for making enzymes. **Enzymes** take one substance, add what are called **cofactors** (such as minerals, energy in the form of ATP, or B vitamins), and makes something brand new. This process takes substance A and turns it into substance B with the use of cofactors. That's how the fats, carbs, and proteins we eat, the water we drink, the air we breathe, and the sunlight we are exposed to turns into or affects something in our body. It is an amazing process.

If you use up all your cofactors, all your energy, you can't keep your genes doing their job. Then you'll find yourself either low in the good things you need to function, or with toxic substances that are not cleared properly and end up hurting you.

Over the past few years, I've become more and more fascinated with how nutrition and environment influence the gene expression. This chapter may contain the most difficult concepts in this book to explain. I'll try to make them easier to understand. Let's start with defining some terms.

Epigenetics is the study of how genetic traits can change and be passed down from generation to generation. Epigenetics often refers to changes in chromosomes that affect gene activity and expression, usually resulting from external or environmental factors. **Genomics** is the branch of molecular biology concerned with the structure, function, evolution, and mapping of genomes. **Nutrigenomics** blends nutrition and genomics. It is the scientific study of the interaction of nutrition and genes, especially with regard to the prevention or treatment of disease. **Proteomics** is the study of proteins. All of our body's functions require proteins and enzymes.

As a nurse practitioner, I am most interested in nutrigenomics, because that is what we can change and alter to provide you the support you need to be as healthy as possible. Unfortunately we can't change the genetics you inherited, but we can teach you how to avoid environmental factors that can impact your weakened genetics, and how lifestyle and nutrition, among other things, can help you compensate for your inherited weakness.

Your **genome** is your complete set of genetic instructions required for you to grow and develop. Your human genome is made up of 3.2 billion base pairs of DNA, twenty-two paired chromosomes, and one X chromosome—with men having one Y chromosome as well, and women having an additional X chromosome. **Deoxyribonucleic acid (DNA)** is the long molecule that contains your unique genetic code. It holds the instructions for making all the proteins in your body. The four main building blocks or bases making

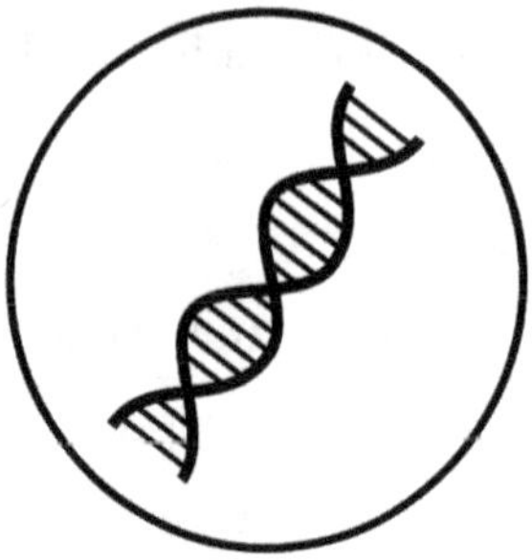

your DNA are **adenine** (A), **cytosine** (C), **guanine** (G), and **thymine** (T). DNA is a double-stranded molecule forming a "double helix" shape, often compared to what a twisted ladder would look like. Each strand of the ladder is paired with a building block. The exact order of these blocks makes you unique. The A should always pair with T, and C with G. Single-stranded DNA coils into threadlike structures called **chromosomes**, which live in the nucleus (middle) of each cell. Each of our twenty-three chromosomes is read to form several small segments, our individual genes. Our cells read this DNA in groups of three bases. Each group of three forms an **amino acid**. Twenty different amino acids exist. Amino acids are often called the "building blocks of life." They can combine in different ways to make proteins needed to make cells, which make up tissues, which make up organs, which make up—us. DNA tells the amino acids how to combine.

When the body wants to turn an action on or off, it uses enzymes. **Enzymes** are protein molecules that catalyze chemical reactions and require cofactors (often metals or vitamin derivatives). Think of enzymes as the workers in the cell. They work on a substrate. Their job as *promotors* is often to make chemical reactions work faster. They take orders to do things like add a methyl group (methylation). *Inhibitors* can turn enzymes off, preventing them from working on the substrate. One example of an inhibitor is the dangerous peroxynitrite free radical. Peroxynitrite can damage our protein and DNA. This inhibits the CBS gene from working properly. In chapter 4, I discuss how cofactors help the enzymes. B6 is a cofactor for CBS.

DNA is our pattern, our blueprint, that tells our cells how to make proteins, essentially telling us how to live (Miller 2015).

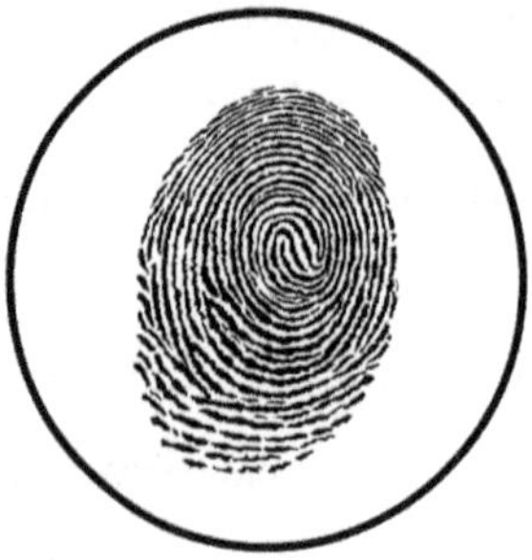

Everyone has their own DNA sequence. That is why people can be identified using DNA fingerprinting.

A **single nucleotide polymorphism** (SNP) is a "swap" at the middle portion of the gene ladder. That swap is a change; it's irregular and not normal. SNPs are what I refer to in this chapter as genetic variants. "**Alleles** are forms of the same gene with small differences in their sequence of DNA bases" (National Institutes of Health 2017). Think of alleles as being one or two versions of a gene that is expressed. One side of the DNA ladder comes from the mother, and the other comes from the father, so each individual inherits two alleles from each gene—one from each parent. If these two alleles are the same, the individual is said to be **homozygous** for that gene. If the alleles are different, they are said to be **heterozygous**. In other words, if you inherit two variants, or defects, you are said to be homozygous for that gene. If you inherit one, you are said to be heterozygous. This can become very confusing, as SNPs can lead to slower or faster enzyme function. SNPs make up our genetic inheritance, and can predispose one to cancer, diabetes, cardiovascular diseases, and even neurological diseases. You may have heard the term **carrier**, which means that you have inherited one bad copy—that you have that SNP.

Some SNPs account for traits as simple as eye color, while others can impact the production of enzymes, impairing that gene function. Despite each individual human's differences, less than 1 percent of total genes vary from person to person.

POLYMORPHISM (SNP)

"Poly" many | **"morphe"** form

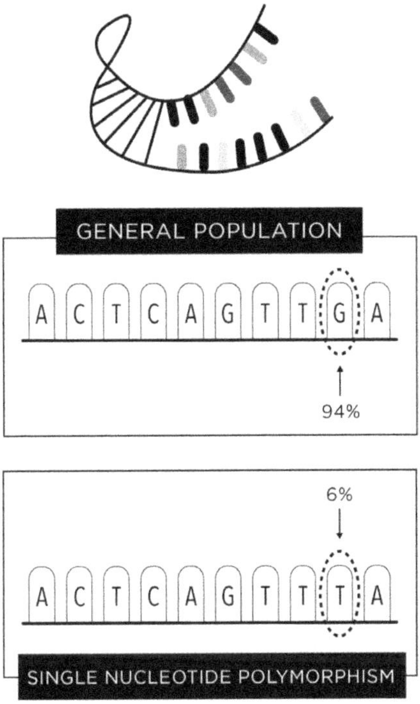

Genes are responsible for how our metabolism works, how we process medications, and even our personalities. Genes control how you clear toxins, and how you neutralize free radicals. They also tell if you are likely to develop a minor or even severe disease.

Genetic testing now allows us to know what diseases we are more likely to contract. It helps provide predictive medicine. It's important to know your genetic variants so you can optimize pregnancy, identify areas of potential nutrient deficiencies (and replete them to help prevent chronic disease), and identify whether you might respond well or poorly to certain natural and pharmaceutical treatments. Everyone wants to feel well. I have a particular interest in looking at SNPs that influence neurotransmitter production, since I've seen so many patients with depression and anxiety. There are thousands to study; choose a few and start learning! Brandon Colby, MD, suggests in his book, *Outsmart Your Genetics*, that knowing our genetic variants may help us avoid our current genetic destiny (Colby 2010).

> **Knowing our genetic variants may help us avoid our current genetic destiny.**

GENETIC TESTING

Genetic screening refers to the genetic testing or analysis that is conducted to evaluate your personal carrier status and risk for diseases. Some companies test for ancestral information, but we won't discuss that in this chapter.

Of the companies that offer genetic testing, I've found it easiest to use 23andme.com. Some require health care providers to authorize the testing ordered, while others allow patients to order directly from the internet. They all test various numbers of SNPs. Every company is different. Some companies only assess for one variant per disease, while others assess for many. You want to verify that the lab performing your testing is CLIA certified, or ISO-15189 accredited.

For years, couples undergoing in vitro fertilization (IVF) have been offered **pre-implant genetic screening (PGS)**, which is an embryo screening initially designed to screen for rare diseases like Tay-Sachs that can cause suffering and death to newborns. The test is run on the embryos themselves, which can pose some risk to the embryo. It has now been expanded to test for other chromosomal diseases, such as Down and Turner syndromes. If couples conceive naturally, they can still undergo PGS between the tenth and thirteenth week. However, this involves a needle being inserted into the womb, which poses risk of miscarriage. Prior to conception, you can pursue genetic testing, which is less invasive, to see if you as a parent are a carrier for these diseases.

Various companies exist that can test for certain panels if you are only interested in your cardiovascular risk, or Alzheimer's risk. What about Huntington's, sickle cell anemia, cystic fibrosis, and muscular dystrophy? These can all be tested for. The list goes on and on. I can't cover them all. However, if you have a family member with a specific genetic condition and you want to be tested only for that genetic variation, several labs can offer you that particular testing. Until recently, genetic testing has been enormously expensive. Now, testing for genetic variants has become available to nearly everyone interested—on average costing less than a nice new pair of shoes, or new golf club.

Several companies now offer an easy, noninvasive cheek swab or saliva test, which can be done in the convenience of your home. The testing is cheapest for my patients to order online through www.23andme.com.

With completion of the testing, you also receive information about ancestry, and many companies specifically advertise this information. In my practice, however, what we are most interested in is the "raw data." Once processed, patients can share their raw data with providers of choice. **Genetic analysis** means interpreting that data. For that, you will need access to an interpretation system and a medical provider who can interpret the data. You can also take your raw data and upload it into various websites like Genetic Genie, LiveWello, MTHFR Support, or Ben Lynch's new interpretation site, StrateGene, to get your genetic analysis report. I often use Bob Miller's MethylGenetic Nutritional Analysis, found at www.dnasupplementation.com.

The benefit of having a provider interpret the data is that they often have access to larger interpretation sites. At my clinic, the site we primarily use is not available to patients. It is a clinician-only site that provides hundreds of more genetic variants than most sites available to patients. Also, even if the patient obtains an interpretation report, they often don't know what to do with the report, or what it means.

I commonly review genetic interpretation reports with my patients, combining this information with their most recent nutritional evaluation. Then I can see not only what predicted nutrients they need based on genetics, but I can also see what nutrients the patient needs on a current functional test. For instance, just because a patient has vitamin D receptor issues doesn't mean they need to take more vitamin D. Testing the level is more important in this case. A patient could have MTHFR variants but might not actually need more folate, too.

Patients often get hung up on this one genetic variant while there are hundreds more that should all be assessed at the same time. In my practice, I don't specialize in testing for disease-specific genes like a gene for Huntington's. Instead, I look at genes that impact your ability to make antioxidants; important nutrients like B12, folate, and choline—genes that support the removal of toxic substances like ammonia and dangerous chemicals.

As I mentioned before, there are genes that are often mutated in people with cancer, but not everyone with those genetic defects gets cancer. Leading researchers believe that environmental factors or other genetic factors that either create more free radicals or inhibit antioxidant production may be the triggers for the health challenge.

For example, the NutriGenetic Research Institute recently found that those with chronic Lyme disease had more genetic variants that would cause iron in the body to create free radicals, and they had less of an ability to make the antioxidants that would neutralize them. If an individual with this genetic pattern also has exposure to toxic chemicals or mold, they may be more likely to have chronic illness.

I believe every specialty subset in medicine will one day test for genetic variants specific to the organ system they treat. This may sound futuristic, but I believe it's realistic!

There are also some specific companies that focus on genetic variants specifically for mental health. Two of those companies are Genomind and Genesight. These companies look at a few variants of genes specific to metabolizing mental health drugs. Each patient report includes a drug interaction summary, which can serve as a guide for clinicians to help determine which therapies may be the least and the most beneficial for the patient. Many insurance companies cover this testing.

For instance, **SLC6A4** is one of the most studied genes in psychiatry. Having this genetic variant suggests that caution should be used with both selective serotonin reuptake inhibitors (SSRIs) and selective norepinephrine reuptake inhibitors (SNRIs). I have had several patients present to my clinic after having tried handfuls of mental health drugs, never having found a great fit and consequently never having achieved relief from their symptoms. Working these individuals through the Longevity Blueprint has reduced their need for medication. When medication is still needed, this type of testing helps to personalize their care and better their success.

GENETICS AND YOU

Another benefit to genetic testing is in determining whether or not you are a carrier. Did you know you could be a carrier for a serious disease? This is called recessive disease state. Even though you may not experience negative symptoms, you can still pass the disease on to the next generation. You may want to know the risk of passing disease on to your children, or you may not.

What if we could predict risk of vaccine injury based on genes? We know enzymes help us process the toxic substances found in vaccines, like mercury and aluminum (Hamborsky, Kroger, and Wolfe 2015). What if you knew your child had several variants suggesting they were not programmed to detox well? Would you be more likely to feed them organic (no pesticides) and vaccinate them more slowly?

Understanding genetic variants might also be particularly more useful to my generation than to the last. My generation—those of us who grew up after the rise of the technology era—has been bombarded with more electromagnetic chaos from technology than the generations that came before us, and from a younger age. Look at school-age children now, who are being exposed to Wi-Fi before they're even in preschool. We now have the largest burden of pesticides, herbicides, and genetically modified foods (GMOs). Many of us have mercury in our mouths, and have been exposed to chemicals and industrial toxins in our personal care products, at our jobs, and maybe even in the womb; we've been exposed to the highest amount of vaccines, and we are the most stressed out any generation has been. Our toxic environment now has a bigger impact on our genes than ever before. As Bob Miller from NutriGenetic Research Institute states, "In all likelihood, those with the weakest genetics unfortunately get impacted first … the worst!"

Testing tells you where your predispositions are. Maybe you need more glutathione? If you know you've inherited several genetic variants for glutathione, the master antioxidant and detoxifier, then you know that you likely don't detox well, so you would know not to expose yourself to toxins on a daily basis. You may consider changing your occupation from painting or welding to something with less toxic exposure.

If you knew you inherited several genetic variants for poor histamine breakdown, you could then choose to avoid foods high in histamine. Can you see how lifestyle becomes so important?

Some of us inherit one or two bad copies of a gene, which means we are already set up for poor enzyme function. Add to this poor gut health and malabsorption of nutrients leading to nutritional deficiencies, and you may have even worse enzyme function, since you don't have the fuel—the cofactors—for that enzyme to work. Genetic testing is a way to find out if there is something important you need that you may not be making enough of. We can then test for that nutrient to confirm your need and give it to you. Isn't that a brilliant concept?

What if you knew you had a **SLC01B1** variant, and you were told that not only would statin medications for cholesterol *not* benefit you, but that they would also cause muscle pain? Would you take the statin? Adverse reactions to properly prescribed medications cause over a hundred thousand deaths every year (USFDA 2016). I can't help but believe many of these could be prevented if we were using our genetic data. Testing is even important for those who feel they are fairly healthy. There are genes for early onset death from heart attack, and genes for reactions to anesthesia.

I know many smokers who are able to consume enormous amounts of caffeine and go right to sleep. It seems unfair. However, our bodies use **CYP1A2** to break down poisons. Smoking turns on this gene, so those who smoke can often tolerate more caffeine, because they have this enzyme active to help break it down.

When I took my fellowship program, the **SIRT1** gene was a highlighted topic. It has been known as an antiaging gene, as it helps us become more stress resistant by delaying cell destruction that results from stress, allowing our cells to repair. This gene is influenced by resveratrol, making it a thousand times more potent. If you had these variants, would you be more likely to take the supplement?

Also, keep in mind that various biomarkers that will indicate the presence of disease can be tested for. If you have strong genetic predispositions, additional labs can be run to confirm or rule out the presence of disease. For instance, as mentioned in chapter 1, someone with HLA DQ2 and HLA DQ8 genotypes may be genetically programmed for gluten sensitivity and celiac disease. Those individuals can then be tested for food sensitivities and celiac for confirmation. However, others feel empowered to know their genes and may still choose to avoid gluten regardless of further testing.

According to Dr. Ritchie Shoemaker's research—which we'll discuss more in chapter 8—almost a quarter of the normal population is genetically susceptible to illness from water damaged buildings, while three-fourths of the population is not. Individuals with these genes, when exposed to biotoxins (like those from mold), can't clear them appropriately. If you knew you were genetically susceptible, would you be more aware of the buildings you entered that could have water damage and mold toxins? Genes can even predict how well you would tolerate food sources high in histamine, tryptophan, tyramine, sulfites, and even sulfur. Again, there are thousands of SNPs that we could discuss. To learn more, check out Ben Lynch's 2018 book *Dirty Genes*.

INDIVIDUAL GENETIC VARIANTS

Thousands of genetic variants exist; over six thousand rare disorders exist. Some are known to have great clinical relevance, and little is known about others. Research on genetic expression is ever emerging, ever changing. Ben Lynch, ND, has helped to lead the charge to discover what genes are most clinically relevant, and how we can optimize them. You can follow him at www.seekinghealth.org.

The following is a brief discussion of only a few clinically relevant genetic variants, some of which are specific to me.

To understand how best to make lifestyle modifications and supplementation in order to support inherited genetics, various pathways need to be studied. Some of these pathways include methylation, transulfuration, methionine, folate, biopterin, kyurenine, arginine, pyruvate, and histamine pathways, to name a few. Finding a functional medicine provider trained in nutrigenomics and these pathways should help you interpret these variants. If you are interested in learning more about genes, classes are available through the MethylGenetic Nutrition website.

In the rest of this chapter, I'll discuss the following genes that are relevant today: VDR, ABP1, SOD2, SOD3, CAT, PON1, MTHFR, GSS, GSR, COMT, CBS, GAD1, BHMT, and GAMT.

Vitamin D Receptor (VDR)

If you have a **vitamin D receptor (VDR)** variant, your need to supplement may be higher. Having low vitamin D can lead to many chronic diseases. The best way to know if you are vitamin D deficient is having your levels tested before supplementing, and then being retested after supplementing to confirm that your levels have improved.

ABP1

ABP1 is the gene that makes the **DAO enzyme** mentioned in chapter 1, which helps to degrade or break down histamine. If you have ABP1 variants combined with **HNMT** variants—which produce the enzyme that uses a methyl group to degrade histamine in the body—you likely will have high histamine and high zonulin (a protein that affects stomach cell wall permeability).

Several genetic variants can predispose an individual to poor detoxification, including SOD2, SOD3, CAT, and PON1.

SOD2, SOD3, and CAT

SOD2 genes make **superoxise dismutase (SOD)** inside of cells, whereas **SOD3** makes it outside of cells. SOD turns the free radical superoxide into H_2O_2 (hydrogen peroxide), which is then turned into water and oxygen by glutathione and catalase. If that process doesn't occur—that is, if SOD doesn't neutralize the free radicals—the free radicals can combine with nitric oxide and create the dangerous oxidizing agent peroxynitrite. Having these variants reduces SOD, and can potentially increase oxidative stress. That can lead to damaged proteins, molecules, and genes within the body, and can eventually lead to chronic diseases like cardiovascular disease. Remember that oxidative stress ages you. When oxidative stress occurs, your cells can literally die. Studies have shown that high oxidative stress can lead to gray hair. Patients with oxidative stress often have low glutathione. The **CAT** gene instructs our bodies to make an enzyme called catalase. **Catalase** is a key antioxidant enzyme in the body's defense against oxidative stress. Variants increase an individual's oxidative stress. Individuals with oxidative stress can benefit from taking antioxidants, specifically SOD and catalase.

Catalase, along with glutathione, is also involved in breaking down hydrogen peroxide. If an individual has some genetic issues that cause iron and/or copper to be out of balance, these minerals can combine with the hydrogen peroxide and create very dangerous hydroxyl radicals, which can do quite a bit of harm.

PON1

Some genes can tell if an individual can't clear herbicides and pesticides well. I've actually had a few patients who had every single **Paraoxonase 1 (PON1)** variant. One young woman felt like she was reacting or detoxing every time she ate, when the foods in fact weren't the problem—the pesticides were. She will need to eat organic the rest of her life. **PON1** protects you against organophosphates (pesticides), helping you detoxify them. This activity is low in newborns, meaning that they are more susceptible to pesticides and thus should be fed organic. If you have several PON1 variants, your ability to detoxify from pesticides may not be optimal. Selenium, vitamins C and E, resveratrol, blueberries, curcumin, and pomegranate are natural agents to promote this gene. Low selenium, high organophosphates like Roundup, lead, and mercury inhibit this gene. It has been associated with ADHD, ALS, autism, and Alzheimer's disease (Lynch 2014).

MTHFR

Methylation (adding a methyl CH_3 group to another molecule) helps regulate gene expression, build neurotransmitters, process chemicals and toxins, produce energy, and reduce the amino acid homocysteine. Methylation variants like **methylenetetrahydrofolate reductase (MTHFR)** SNPs may be very important for many reasons. The MTHFR gene provides instructions for making the methylenetetrahydrofolate reductase enzyme, which is required for the body to convert homocysteine to methionine. The more MTHFR variants you have, the greater likelihood your enzyme function is very impaired, which means you can't convert homocysteine to methionine. Thus, homocysteine can build up, increasing cardiovascular risk.

The top two commonly seen variations are A1298C and C677T. We are seeing more of these variations and we are also seeing more infertility and autism. Could there be an association here? This variant is also associated with mental illness, addictions, cancer, and cardiovascular disease-related deaths. MTHFR is the predominant enzyme that converts folic acid/folate to its active form (methylfolate) needed for synthesis of serotonin, dopamine, and norepinephrine. It's possible that fortifying foods with folic acid has been very dangerous for these individuals. Folic acid is not helpful, because these individuals can't utilize it. In fact, it attaches itself to the same receptor in the body used to absorb folate, so it basically further reduces folate status. These individuals need actual folate found in nature—not folic acid, which is synthetic.

It has been proven that folate status during pregnancy is crucial to the development of the child. Recommendations for 400 mcg folic acid were created based on the average woman with average genes. Women of childbearing years with genetic variants A1298C and C677T should avoid folic acid and instead take methylfolate or folate. You may need 1,000 to 4,000 mcg or even more, pending your levels. MTHFR has also been associated with tongue and lip ties, and, as in Chelsea's case, her miscarriages. MTHFR variants have been associated with increased risk for blood clots. Pregnancy alone increases risks of blood clots. Chelsea had high homocysteine and MTHFR variants. Her baby could have been miscarried due to little clots reducing circulation to the baby. Chelsea was placed on methylfolate supplementation and Lovenox injections to keep her blood thin through her pregnancy, and it was successful. She has now delivered a healthy baby girl!

Do you have newly discovered MTHFR variants? Check out Ben Lynch's site, MTHFR.net, which contains his suggested protocols for both top variants. Unfortunately, many people do genetic testing on their own, run it through online software, find they have MTHFR genetic variants, and then order the methylfolate products. It's not unusual to have a positive response for a short period of time, followed by either anxiety or inflammation. That is because folate can turn into an excitatory neurotransmitter called glutamate, or through other pathways, it can lower glutamate and cause inflammation.

We are learning that it's usually best to make sure glutamate and glutathione are at optimal levels before supplementing with folate. That's why working with an experienced health provider is often your best bet, before you take matters into your own hands.

The ongoing research regarding MTHFR is often very overwhelming for my patients. I have narrowed these protocols down and simplified them, as many clinicians do. I typically order a comprehensive nutritional assessment for patients. If low on B12 and B9, I place my patients on hydroxyl or methylcobalamin and methylfolate. However, I recommend they avoid folic acid. I often verify they are on curcumin, multivitamin, vitamin D, fish oil, and probiotics. And again, optimizing glutathione levels first is important. This can be accomplished using N-acetylcysteine and or glutathione.

I also recommend testing them for food sensitivities, or at least that they stop consuming dairy and gluten. I always recommend they eat organic and work to start detoxing, using an infrared sauna, drinking filtered water, using a home air filter, and considering a liver detox program. I also often order a homocysteine level. If found to be high, recommended homocysteine-lowering nutrients include methyl and hydroxycobalamin, methylfolate, trimethylglycine, riboflavin (B2), pyridoxine (B6), and phosphatidylcholine.

Urine hormone testing for estrogen metabolism also shows methylation of estrogens. Read more about this in chapter 6. I typically presume that if methylation of estrogens is optimal, it may indeed be optimal for other toxins. If it is poor, then likely methylation elsewhere is also poor.

For a true methylation assessment, I use Health Diagnostics and Research Institute (www.hdri-usa.com). I often order a baseline assessment, and then reorder the methylation panel eight weeks after beginning supplementation protocol.

GSS, GSR

The major glutathione genes are **glutathione synthetase (GSS)** and **glutathione reductase (GSR)**. Further discussed in chapter 4, glutathione is a powerful antioxidant that helps to neutralize free radicals and prevent their formation. Those with low glutathione can have poor detoxification. Individuals with low glutathione often report sensitivities to smells. Glutathione recharges other antioxidants like vitamins C and E. Glutathione has the ability to recycle itself via the enzyme glutathione reductase (GSR).

There are also numerous genes associated with production and degradation of neurotransmitters, which are like chemical messengers. Some of these genes are histamine, serotonin, GABA, glutamate, dopamine, epinephrine, and norepinephrine, though the gene COMT is the most studied. I will also briefly discuss the genes CBS, GAD1, BHMT, and GAMT.

COMT

The **COMT** gene provides instructions for making the enzyme **catechol-O-methyltransferase**, which helps to degrade or break down excitatory neurotransmitters and catecholamines such as dopamine, epinephrine, and norepinephrine, also known as adrenaline. As with many genetic variants, the more variants and combinations with other problematic variants there are, the greater the chances of a large problem. Being homozygous (having inherited two bad copies) for both COMT V158M and COMT H62H can create a storm of adrenaline. These individuals have issues breaking down epinephrine, norepinephrine, dopamine, and estrogens. They often tend to have high cortisol, and their response to stimulants is magnified. I am homozygous for both of these COMT variants. I can't tolerate any stimulants. I can't even sip caffeine without getting palpitations and anxiety. Sometimes these individuals also cannot tolerate methyl B12, methylfolate, or trimethylglycine. Magnesium is COMT's biggest cofactor. Since I have inherited major variations here, I load up on what should help support these genes. I take LB's Magnesium Chelate religiously. S-adenosyl methionine (SAM-e) is another cofactor here. If very anxious, niacin may be able to help these individuals reduce their adrenaline, as it lowers methyl groups. These individuals can experience heavy periods, PMS, and poor estrogen clearance, potentially increasing risk for breast cancer. These individuals should have their estrogen metabolism assessed. Additionally, not just treating the gene, but also assessing the patient and discovering what other genetic variants the individual has will help personalize their treatment. On a positive note, I was happy to discover that there can also be benefits to these genetic variants, like "improved working memory, executive function and higher IQ" (Rhonda 2013).

CBS

Cystathionine beta synthase (CBS) allows homocysteine to move down the transsulfuration pathway. Having CBS variants could cause homocysteine to travel too fast, stressing the SUOX enzyme and leading to excess glutamate, which can then trigger anxiety and stress. Checking urine sulfite levels can help provide insight into whether this is happening. The major cofactor for CBS is pyridoxol 5 phosphate (B6). This is also promoted by SAM-e.

GAD1

Glutamate decarboxylase 1 (**GAD1**) is needed to convert the excitotoxin glutamate into the calming neurotransmitter **GABA**. Homozygous individuals feel this stress more than do heterozygous individuals. I have this genetic variant, which predisposes me to feeling more anxiety. I can't tolerate any foods with monosodium glutamate (MSG) or else I have heart palpitations, flushing, and dizziness. Many heroin users and alcoholics have this gene and don't convert their glutamate into GABA well. Guess what boosts GABA? Heroine and alcohol. Magnesium and B6 are necessary cofactors for this glutamate-to-GABA conversion. I take these every day to help my glutamate convert to GABA. Many individuals with the GAD1 also benefit from taking honokiol, calming amino acids such as L-theanine, or GABA, which help to reduce excitatory glutamate. Supplementing with molybdenum can help to unlock GAD1.

Betaine-homocysteine methyltransferase (**BHMT**) converts betaine and homocysteine to dimethylglycine and methionine. **BHMT** variants slow conversion of homocysteine into methionine and can push it down the transsulfuration pathways, causing high glutamate, anxiety, and high cortisol.

Guanidinoacetate methyltransferase (**GAMT**) is a gene that converts SAM-e into creatine, which helps with muscle strength. At a conference, I once heard a patient testimony about how taking creatine resolved her fibromyalgia. She had never known to try it until she found out that she had this genetic variant.

Factor V Leiden is a mutation of one of the clotting factors in the blood called **factor V**. Having just one bad copy of factor V and being heterozygous increases your risk of having a clotting event in your lifetime. I see this commonly when a patient is on birth control. They experience a blood clot, they get tested for factor V, and their testing returns positive. They stop the birth control, but now they are aware that their risk for clotting is higher. This can also increase risk of miscarriage. If it's determined that you have factor V, ask your provider to also order platelets C-reactive protein and fibrinogen.

Factor II-Prothrombin 20210A

The **factor II** gene provides instructions for your body to make a protein called prothrombin (also called coagulation factor II). The factor II variant is similar to factor V. Again, being heterozygous increases your risk for a clotting event sometime in your life if not monitored. This gene also increases risk for miscarriage—the uterus is fed with capillaries, and if a clot occurs the blood flow there will be altered.

Individuals with factor V and II should not sit for prolonged periods of time and should not smoke. They should, however, exercise, prevent dehydration, and avoid birth control. These disorders can also be managed by taking omega-3 fatty acids (fish oil), which helps to thin the blood. Some individuals require anticoagulation therapy with pharmaceutical agents, as these individuals are at higher risk of developing a deep vein thrombosis (DVT), also known as a clot.

ApoE

Since heart disease is the leading cause of death, genes that influence cardiovascular risk have a huge impact on our longevity. The most common gene affecting cholesterol and CHD disease is the apolipoprotein E, or **ApoE**. This gene is important because it helps determine how your body will respond to alcohol, fat, exercise, and medication. It also helps you repair neurons in the brain when damaged. It helps with your brain synaptic plasticity, which is responsible for learning and memory. If this gene doesn't function well, "harmful deposits can build up, structural integrity of brain cells is compromised and synaptic plasticity may deteriorate" (Colby 2010, 208). You inherit an ApoE2, ApoE3, or ApoE4 gene from each parent. The E4 variant doesn't function well. So, for instance, if you inherited E2 from Mom and E2 from Dad, your genotype would be E2/E2. E2/E2 or E2/E3 places you at 40 percent lower risk for Alzheimer's. If you inherit any E3, this is considered the normal genotype and you are at no greater risk for cardiovascular disease or Alzheimer's. However, if you inherit E4, you are at increased risk for both cardiovascular disease and Alzheimer's. If you inherit E2/E4, you have 160 percent increased risk. If you are E4/E4 you have >1,000 percent increased risk. Combine E4 variants with SORL1 or TOMM40 variants and the risk for Alzheimer's increases further.

Interestingly if you have this E4 genetic variant and you suffer from head injury like a concussion, this increases your risk of Alzheimer's 200 percent. If you knew you had the variant, would you be less likely to play football or hockey?

It has been predicted that by 2029 all baby boomers will be over the age of sixty-five. Alzheimer's affects one in eight people over sixty-five years old, and one in two people over eighty-five. Medicare spends more on Alzheimer's than any other disease. What if we could help those individuals who are most predisposed to Alzheimer's prevent it?

Lifestyle to Optimize Genes

Once we know what genetic variants we possess, we can change our lifestyle to balance or reduce that risk. You may or may not be familiar with the BRCA1 and BRCA2 genes for breast cancer. Individuals with the BRCA1 gene have a 65 percent chance of developing breast cancer. You know what escalates that risk? Having those genes in combination with other genes. Having one genetic variant doesn't predict your future.

We can't change our genetics. As Sharon Moalem, MD, PhD, says in her book, *Inheritance: How Our Genes Change Our Lives—and Our Lives Change Our Genes*, "Our genetic legacy was completely fixed when our parents conceived us" (Moalem 2014). However, although your genes predispose you, the good news is that you can change your lifestyle and environment to influence them for the better.

Everything you do influences your genetic expression. Lack of sleep, poor nutrition, and exposure to toxins all influence your genes.

One of the most powerful lifestyle interventions we have is our decision to reduce our toxic load. Chapter 5 is entirely dedicated to the importance of detoxing, which will help influence all your genes for the better. Radiation from x-rays and even flying in an airplane affects us on a cellular level. Electromagnetic chaos from the computer I'm using to write this book does the same thing.

High-quality, nutrient-dense food is the best fuel for our genes. Chemicals like pesticides and herbicides on nonorganic foods contribute to our toxic load.

Nutritional deficiencies, excess inflammation, infections, and how you were taken care of early in life all influence your genome and eventually its expression. Choices like consuming alcohol and smoking can negatively impact our gene expression. Heavy metals from our personal care products and fillings in our teeth also work against us.

If you knew you had a lung cancer gene increasing your risk for lung cancer, would that help you quit smoking? If you knew you had the "obesity" genes, would you frequent McDonald's less often and the gym more? If you had a gene predisposing you to heart arrhythmias, blood clots, or stroke, would you frequent the gym more often and be less likely to sit for extended periods of time?

It is very important to establish proper sleep patterns to allow your body time to repair and heal. Managing your stress is likely the most important recommendation for optimizing your genetics. Your negative thoughts can do a lot of damage, while your positive thoughts can promote healing.

How important is lifestyle? Changing the genetic expression can be the difference between a lesion remaining noncancerous and becoming cancerous.

Working through the Longevity Blueprint will help you optimize your genes. The basic recommendations for keeping those good genes turned on and bad genes turned off are mentioned throughout this book—they are not confined to this chapter alone.

Nutrients to Optimize Genetics

I've had patients present me with their genetic reports on their first visit, expecting an easy fix and basic supplement recommendations. I often recommend LB Mitochondrial Complex with nutrients and antioxidants to feed the mitochondria. However, treating each patient is actually more complex than that.

I don't typically start with genetic testing for any patient. As the Longevity Blueprint recommends, I always start by optimizing gut health in my patients, and then fixing nutritional deficiencies. Remember, nutritional testing shows not just what someone is predisposed to being low in, but what they are actually low in.

As will be discussed in chapter 5, getting toxins out of your life is highly recommended in order to limit the burden on your genes. Get tested to see what nutrients you need to optimize your genetics.

As Terry Wahls, MD, says in his book, *The Wahls Protocol*, "Through optimal lifestyle choices you can keep the most harmful genes in the 'off' position and the most health-promoting genes in the 'on' position" (Wahls 2014).

CONCLUSION

Chelsea and her husband from earlier in the chapter were found to both be heterozygous for MTHFR A1298C. After her MTHFR variants were discovered and she received anticoagulation support she was able to carry a baby to full term. She continues to thank our clinic for discovering this variant, making her family whole by allowing her to fulfill her dream of having a baby.

I hope and believe the future of medicine will incorporate genetics. Can you imagine if your doctor knew what drugs you should and shouldn't take based on your genes? This is truly how we should be personalizing health care. Knowledge is power, right? You and your medical provider can use your genetic information to help you make the best decisions regarding how you live your life—from what you eat to how often you undergo a liver detox program. The celebrity Angelina Jolie even took her findings to the next step and had an entire hysterectomy and mastectomy.

Genes influence longevity. Can you imagine not having electricity in your home? Would you neglect your power if it went out? It's important to value your genetics much more than you value the electricity in your home. When the variants pile up, they create inflammation. Testing for several variants provides greater benefit to better assess risk. Looking at one SNP can be disastrous, invoking unnecessary fears. You've got to look at patterns.

So where do you start? Find a provider familiar with nutrigenomics. Several patients have sought me out simply because I am listed as a provider familiar with this testing, one of the few providers in Iowa listed in the online Seeking Health directory located at seekinghealth.org. At that site, you can search the physician directory for providers near you who have taken Ben Lynch's certification courses in genetics.

Genetic counselors are available in most larger cities. You can find one at www.nsgc.org.

Meeting with a genetic counselor can significantly reduce psychological stress, but keep in mind that not all of these counselors are trained in nutrition. If you are a provider, consider attending a Seeking Health conference, or a MethylGenetic Nutrition conference. I continue to be amazed at how much I learn every time I attend.

You must be prepared for what your testing may reveal. Ask yourself if you really want to know if you are predisposed to certain diseases. There's no reason to test if you aren't going to do anything with the results. If you want to know, as Colby says, we can then work to "outsmart our genes" (Colby 2010).

Remember that genetics is only one piece of the puzzle—one piece of your blueprint, one piece of your destiny—but your DNA doesn't have to be your destiny. Genetics load the gun, but lifestyle and environment pull the trigger. That means you have the power to make a difference before it's too late. As Moalem says, "Your behavior can and does dictate your genetic destiny" (Moalem 2014, 30). You can't change the wiring in your house, but you can turn that electricity on and off. We can't change our genetics, but we can change our genetic expression. "How you choose to live will determine how well you treat your genome" (Moalem 2014, 174).

You can optimize your genetics by following your Longevity Blueprint.

Remember that genetics is only one piece of the puzzle—one piece of your blueprint, one piece of your destiny—but your DNA doesn't have to be your destiny. Genetics load the gun, but lifestyle and environment pull the trigger.

You can't change the wiring in your house, but you can turn that electricity on and off. We can't change our genetics, but we can change our genetic expression.

Longevity Blueprint Nutraceutical Products

Here are my favorite Longevity Blueprint nutrients to influence genetics.

- Methyl B Complex

- SL Methyl Bs
- Magnesium Chelate
- Mitochondrial Complex

Chapter 3 Resources

23andme: www.23andme.com

Genetic Genie: http://geneticgenie.org/

Genesight: https://genesight.com/

Genomind: https://genomind.com/

Live Wello: https://livewello.com/

MethylGenetic Nutrition: http://www.methylgeneticnutritionclasses.com/

www.dnasupplementation.com (for health professionals only)

MTHFR Support: https://mthfrsupport.com/

National Society of Genetic Counselors: http://www.nsgc.org

Strategene: https://seekinghealth.org/product/strategene/

Seeking Health Physician Directory: https://seekinghealth.org/

Chapter 3 References

1. Colby, Brandon. *Outsmart Your Genes.* New York: Penguin Group, 2010.
2. Hamborsky, Jennifer, Andrew Kroger, and Charles Wolfe. *Epidemiology and Prevention of Vaccine-Preventable Diseases.* The Communication and Education Branch, National Center for Immunization and Respiratory Diseases, Centers for Disease Control and Prevention, (April 2015). https://www.cdc.gov/vaccines/pubs/pinkbook/downloads/table-of-contents.pdf.
3. Lynch, Ben. *Dirty Genes.* New York: HarperCollins, 2018.

4. Lynch, Ben. *Methylation and Clinical Nutrigenomics* pt. 2. Online seminar, https://www.drbenlynch.com/product/methylation-clinical-nutrigenomics-part-2.

5. Miller, B. *Methylgenetic Nutrition*. Online certification course, module 1, http://nutrigeneticresearch.talentlms.com/catalog/info/id:130.

6. Moalem, Sharon. *Inheritance. How Our Genes Change Our Lives and Our Lives Change Our Genes*. New York: Hachette Book Group, 2014.

7. Genetics Home Reference. National Institutes of Health. US National Library of Medicine. Retrieved March 2017. https://ghr.nlm.nih.gov/.

8. Rhonda (no last name given). "Understand COMT and Change Your Life!" Midway Center for Integrative Medicine, February 2013, http://www.themidwaycenter.com/understand-comt-and-change-your-life/.

9. US Food & Drug Administration. "Preventable Adverse Drug Reactions: A Focus on Drug Interactions." US Department of Health and Human Services (2016). https://www.fda.gov/Drugs/DevelopmentApprovalProcess/DevelopmentResources/DrugInteractionsLabeling/ucm110632.htm

10. Wahls, T. *The Wahls Protocol: A Radical New Way to Treat All Chronic Autoimmune Conditions Using Paleo Principles.* New York: Avery, 2014.

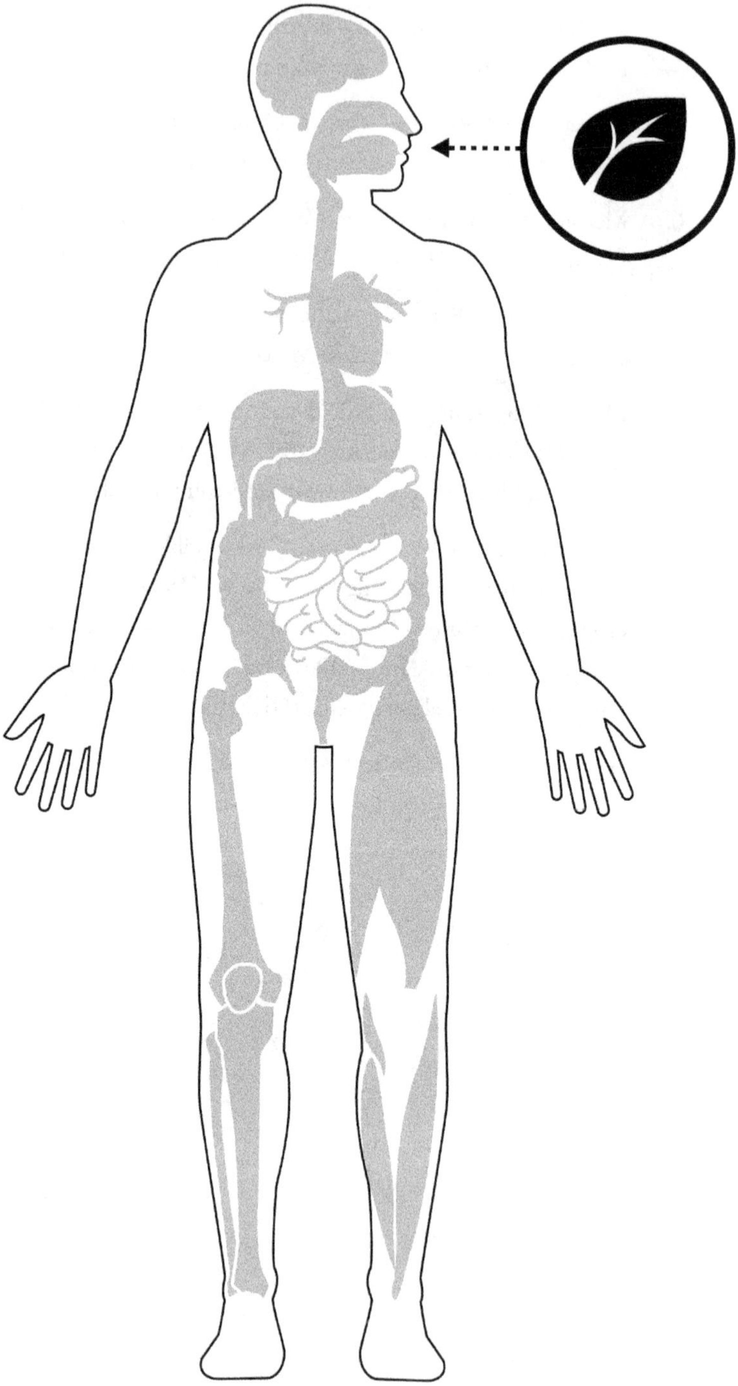

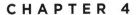

CHAPTER 4

HAVING THE KEYS TO UNLOCK DOORWAYS: REPLETING NUTRITIONAL DEFICIENCIES

The doctor of the future will give no medicines, but will interest his patients in the care of the human frame, in diet, and in the cause and prevention of disease.

—Thomas Edison

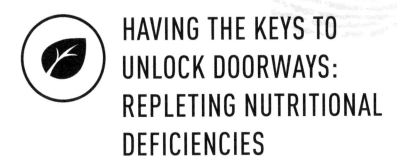

Kate was seventy years old and had osteoporosis, but she ate organic and still exercised five days each week. She slept well. She had no major symptoms. She took only one medication for reflux, omeprazole. She detoxed twice each year. Her hormones were balanced. She was really an ideal patient. She took a "one-a-day" multivitamin and a salmon oil product. Because she'd made wise lifestyle choices, she was shocked with the results of her nutrient testing. She thought that because of the choices she made on a daily basis, she wouldn't need to heavily supplement. She was partially correct. Her lifestyle choices made her less dependent on supplements, but her testing still revealed her greatest needs. She didn't realize her digestion wasn't optimal, and that the medication she was taking was blocking acid, disrupting her absorption. She also didn't know that, even though she ate organic, her foods weren't giving her all of what her body needed to function optimally. Not to mention that she was aging, which also increased her needs.

Jared was thirty-five years old and did not eat organic. He ate fast food several times each week. He didn't exercise. He worked overtime every week, and he was in a stressed place when he came to our clinic. He took medications for blood pressure, diabetes, and cholesterol. He wasn't shocked with the results of his nutrient testing. He knew his body was suffering, and he wanted to know what he should be taking to help his body function better. With his poor food choices, Jared was clearly on his way to early death. Because of those choices, he was severely deficient in his nutritional needs, and had a very high need for supplementing.

Although Karen was in better shape than Jared and already making better food choices, both of these patients demonstrate how food choices are an important part of lifestyle for health, and how supplementation is necessary.

Patrick Flynn, DC, has used the example of a wilting plant or flower to explain the importance of nutrition. When you visualize a wilting plant or flower, what do you think it needs? You may argue that it needs a little tender, loving care, but it also needs water, proper soil, nutrients, and sunlight. You don't take a houseplant to the doctor to get recommendations for drugs or surgery. Instead, when you see it wilt, you ask what it needs to be healthy and to grow.

It's the same with the human body. Why do plants need nutrients, anyway? They need nutrients for the same reasons our bodies do. The essential **macronutrients** for life include carbohydrates, proteins (amino acids), and lipids (fats), as well as fiber. Our needed **micronutrients** includes vitamins, minerals, antioxidants, and, of course, lots of water. I mentioned fiber and fats briefly in chapter 1. In this chapter, I'll discuss amino acids, which come from protein, as well as several micronutrients. Humans need nutrients to grow and develop just as plants do.

Obtaining these nutrients is a bit of a choice. You may have heard the comment, "You are what you eat," which is true to some extent. Food choices are very important. Consuming a diet high in sugar and low in fruits and vegetables increases your risk for cardiovascular disease, cancer, and diabetes. These diseases are directly linked to the foods you eat. Processed foods contain more calories, more macronutrients, and fewer micronutrients. When you eat more unprocessed, raw, real foods, you are giving your body more micronutrients. If you want to increase your longevity, you need to be thinking about your nutritional status daily.

The best advice I've read about what to eat and what not to eat was by author Michael Pollen. He says, "Eat food. Not too much, mostly plants" (Pollen 2009). You might not want to hear it, but what you eat has consequences. Read his books if you want to learn how to make the best food choices. I find it comical but true that he writes, "It's not food if it's called by the same name in every language (Big Mac, Cheetos, or Pringles)" (Pollen 2009, 45). He also says, "Eating what stands on one leg (mushrooms and plant foods) is better than eating what stands on two legs (fowl), which is better that

> **What you eat has consequences.**

eating what stands of four legs (cows, pigs, and other mammals)" (Pollen 2009, 55). What he means is to eat mostly plants, which harbor loads of live nutrients.

> **You are not only what you eat—but what it eats, too.**

Remember, you are not only what *you* eat—but what it eats, too. When you eat beef, do you know what the cow you are eating ate? Was it fed grass or corn? If it was fed grass, you reap the benefits of more omega-3s (which are anti-inflammatory) and less omega-6s (which are pro-inflammatory, from corn).

Pollen also advises not to eat too much. Much research exists on caloric restriction extending our lives. Stop eating when you are 70 percent full. Only eat as much as the bowl size you can make by putting your hands together. And, "Eat breakfast as a king, lunch like a prince, and dinner like a pauper" (Pollen 2009, 119). Remember, as Hippocrates said, to "let food be your medicine, and medicine be your food." As I mentioned earlier, Pollen also says that most of us aren't eating what our grandparents and parents ate as children (Pollen 2008). In fact, our grandmothers may not recognize any of the complex processed foods we have at our tables now. He recommends not eating anything your great-grandmother wouldn't recognize as food, like "packaged Go-Gurt."

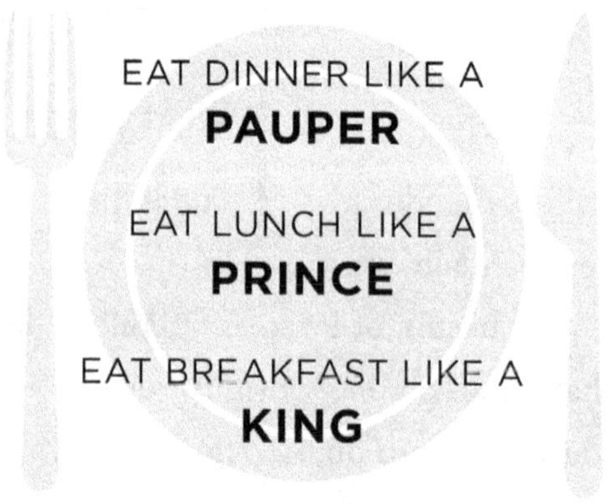
EAT DINNER LIKE A
PAUPER
EAT LUNCH LIKE A
PRINCE
EAT BREAKFAST LIKE A
KING

So how does food help the body? What do nutrients actually do?

Nutrients are involved in a variety of chemical reactions in the body. As Pollen writes, "Foods are essentially the sum of their nutrient parts" (Pollen 2008, 28). In chapter 1, I explained the process of digestion. After food is digested, nutrients are transported through the body to assist in all the metabolic processes that happen in our cells and that are necessary for life. The nutrients transporting themselves throughout your body is a little like moving through the rooms in a house in which each room has a door that is locked. In order to move from room to room, you must have the key to unlock the door.

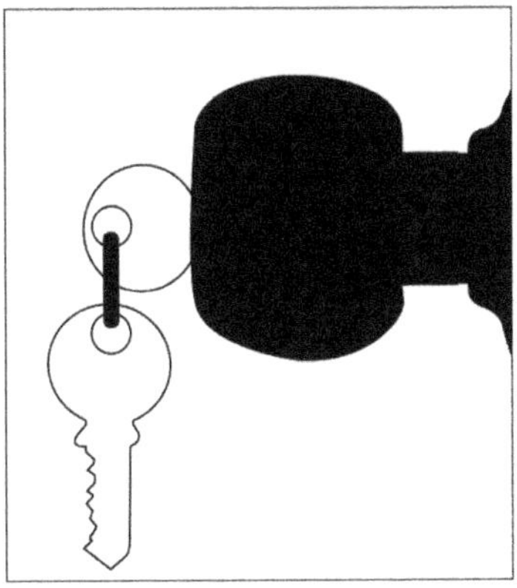

The same is true with your body. Every cell in your body has a receptor site that receptors bind to, like a key fitting into the keyhole. For that receptor to bind/fit correctly, to unlock the door, your body requires all the micronutrients listed in this chapter. As Wahls states, "When the cells aren't getting what they need, the body doesn't work right, and something (usually many somethings) will go wrong somewhere…your mitochondria won't produce energy efficiently and that can eventually launch a chronic disease process" (Wahls 2014, 22–23). Wahls has created what she calls the Wahls protocol in effort to teach individuals how to feed their mitochondria and nurture their cells. This is how she was able to overcome her multiple sclerosis, get out of her wheelchair, and take her life back. For more information visit www.terrywahls.com.

Everyone has inherited good and bad genes. Having the proper balance of the nutrients in this chapter will help keep your genes functioning as they should. The body is composed of billions of cells, groups, enzymes, and systems that work miraculously together, keeping all your body functions processing appropriately. Enzymes are proteins that catalyze a chemical reaction. Some enzymes need helpers or partners.

A cofactor is a non-protein "helper" chemical compound bound to and needed by the protein. Iron and zinc are examples of cofactors. A coenzyme is a non-protein "partner" molecule that carries chemical groups between enzymes. Vitamins are good examples of coenzymes. Cofactors and coenzymes are required for biochemical reactions in our bodies.

DOSING OF NUTRIENTS

What dose of each nutrient do you need every day? The answer varies from person to person and from day to day. The Food and Nutrition Board of the National Academy of Science developed the recommended daily allowance, which you know as the recommended dietary allowances, or RDAs, back in 1943. These recommendations have now turned into the reference dietary intakes (RDI). These guidelines were essentially created around war time when determining exactly what military personnel needed in the form of nutrition. At the time, there were a number of draftee rejections due to vitamin deficiencies.

What's important to note is that these recommendations haven't changed despite our depleted soils, and despite the decline in nutrients in our foods. Also, we now know that our genes influence our need for nutrients, and that genes vary from person to person. The RDI takes none of that into consideration.

It's important to note that the RDIs are the absolute minimum necessary to prevent a deficient state; they are not about promoting health. They essentially mean that you have to take *X* amount of vitamin C to avoid getting scurvy. However, those recommendations are not the doses to truly prevent disease, to replace what your combination of drugs robs you of, to make up for your three cups of coffee per day, or to replete what running a marathon depleted in you.

It's important to note that the RDIs are the absolute minimum necessary to prevent a deficient state; they are not about promoting health.

If you don't have optimal levels of all the nutrients listed in this chapter, you run the risk for chronic disease and cancer. Researchers in the *Journal of the American Medical Association* stated, "Suboptimal vitamin states are associated with many chronic diseases including cardiovascular disease, cancer, and osteoporosis" (Fletcher and Fairfield 2002). RDIs are also based on a two thousand-calorie-per-day diet. How many individuals eating the Standard American Diet (SAD) consume far more calories than that? So, the RDIs are a great place to start; however, most of my patients require much higher doses daily. Remember, "As you feed your cells what they need, your cells will rebuild you" (Wahls 2014).

What follows is only a brief summation of the importance of each cofactor/nutrient. Remember to think of each of these as keys that unlock doors for important reactions in the body. Each listed nutrient has many more functions and accomplishes much more than is listed below. For more information, visit the Linus Pauling Institute at the Oregon State University website, lpi.oregonstate.edu.

There are four groups of essential nutrients that I will discuss next: vitamins, minerals, amino acids, and essential fatty acids. Lastly, I will discuss antioxidants.

Vitamins

Fat-soluble vitamins are stored in the fat cells. They include vitamins A, D, E, and K.

Vitamin A is a generic term that refers to fat-soluble compounds found as *preformed* vitamin A (retinol) in animal products, and as *provitamin* A carotenoids in plants (fruits and vegetables). The three active forms of vitamin A in the body are retinol, retinal, and retinoic acid (LPI 2017). Vitamin A is important for immune function, skin, mucous membranes, and vision. Being low in vitamin A can actually cause night blindness. Also, low vitamin A can inhibit proper thyroid function. I've seen several patients through the years with dry eyes who benefit from vitamin A supplementation. Major food sources include orange veggies like sweet potatoes, pumpkins, tomatoes, carrots, steak, liver, dairy, and eggs. Too much vitamin A can cause liver damage. Higher doses should be taken with caution in pregnant patients, as too much could harm the fetus. The tolerable upper limit in adults is 10,000 IU/day.

Vitamin D is made in the skin upon exposure to sunlight and is then converted through the kidney and liver to its active form, which influences the expression of hundreds of genes (Higdon 2000). Vitamin D is essential for bone and teeth health. It is required for proper calcium absorption, is necessary for blood clotting, and is a potent immune system modulator. Numerous epidemiological studies have demonstrated the importance of higher vitamin D levels.

The lower the levels, the higher the risk for autoimmune diseases like type 1 diabetes, multiple sclerosis, rheumatoid arthritis, and systemic lupus erythematosus. Severe deficiency causes rickets. Vitamin D3 (cholecalciferol) is the superior form that is more easily metabolized by the body. Major food sources of vitamin D are oily fish, dairy, and nuts. Dosing is based on the individual's level. Some patients can maintain optimal levels above 50 on 5,000 IU D3 daily, while others require much higher doses. Oftentimes, when my patients are initially deficient, I place them on a short course of 50,000 IU D3 two to three times a week for fifteen doses, and then recheck the level. Simply taking 1,000 to 2,000 IU D3 a day is not enough to quickly improve the level in a deficient patient.

Vitamin E is actually a name for eight fat-soluble isoforms: α-, β-, γ-, and δ-tocopherol and α-, β-, γ-, and δ-tocotrienol. The body preferentially uses α-tocopherol, making it the best form to take (Higdon 2000). Vitamin E can help reduce hot flashes, prevent chronic diseases and cancer, and improve immune function. Major food sources of vitamin E are nuts and seeds. The typical recommendation is 400 IU daily, although toxicity hasn't been seen in doses up to 3,200 IUs (LPI 2017). Remember, vitamin E can thin the blood. Be cautious if you are already taking other blood thinners.

Vitamin K includes phylloquinone (vitamin K1) and a family of molecules called menaquinones (MKs or vitamin K2). K1 is found in green leafy veggies while K2 is produced by bacteria in the gut. Vitamin K is important for blood clotting. Vitamin K deficiency increases the risk of hemorrhaging (excessively bleeding). Vitamin K is also important for reducing plaque buildup, as well as for reducing chronic disease (Higdon 2000). The average dose of vitamin K2 (as menaquinone-7) offered in my practice is 45 mcg/day.

Water-soluble vitamins are excreted or eliminated by your body and are not stored. They need to be taken every day.

Vitamin B1 is also known as thiamine. Thiamine is involved in several enzyme reactions in the body, including those responsible for the metabolism of carbohydrates and production of energy. Severe thiamine deficiency can lead to beriberi. Beriberi is a disease that affects multiple organ systems—including the central and peripheral nervous systems. Major food sources include fortified grains, wheat germ, nuts, legumes, and peas. The recommended dosage is 10–100 mg daily.

Vitamin B2 is also known as riboflavin and is a precursor of the coenzymes flavin adenine dinucleotide (FAD) and flavin mononucleotide (FMN). FAD and FMN are carriers in reactions involved in metabolic pathways and energy. Vitamin B2 is also very important in working to regenerate glutathione, the most powerful antioxidant in the body. Deficiency can lead to headaches, depression, and cracked skin. Major food sources include brewer's yeast and liver. The recommended dosage is 10–100 mg daily.

Vitamin B3 includes both niacin and nicotinic acid. It is beneficial for lowering cholesterol and triglycerides. Vitamin B3 is important in energy production, since it is used in the metabolism of tryptophan and serotonin. Severe deficiency can lead to a condition known as pellagra, which affects the skin, and to problems with the digestive and nervous systems. Major food sources include meat, cereal, beans, brewer's yeast, rice, and animal organs (such as liver). The recommended dosage is 50–3,000 mg/day. The tolerable upper intake level (UL) for niacin is also based on skin flushing, which is an adverse effect of niacin.

Vitamin B5 is also known as pantothenic acid. It is a precursor in the synthesis of coenzyme A, which is essential to many biochemical reactions that sustain life. It is found nearly everywhere in the body. It is also important for the adrenal glands. Major food sources include animal organs (liver and kidney), fish, shellfish, milk products, eggs, avocados, legumes, mushrooms, and sweet potatoes. The recommended dosage is 50–250 mg/day. Little or no toxicity has been associated with supplementation, and no tolerable upper intake level (UL) has been set.

Vitamin B6's active form is pyridoxal 5'-phosphate (P5P), which is essential to over a hundred enzymes, mostly involved in protein metabolism. It is necessary to convert *all* amino acids. B6 can help to lower homocysteine, which is an independent risk factor for cardiovascular disease. It is also essential in the production of many neurotransmitters. Many people with monosodium glutamate (MSG) sensitivity are deficient in vitamin B6. Deficiency can cause neurologic, mental health symptoms like depression, irritability, insomnia, and confusion. Vitamin B6 is found in a variety of foods, including fish, poultry, nuts, legumes, potatoes, and bananas. The recommended dosage is 30-500 mg daily.

Vitamin B7 is also known as biotin. It can be made by the flora in your gut, and thus taking antibiotics can reduce biotin. Biotin is essential for hair and nail growth. Deficiency can lead to hair loss, cradle cap in newborns, and dermatitis. Biotin helps increase insulin sensitivity and thus can be helpful for diabetics. Major food sources are egg yolk, liver, and yeast. The recommended dosage is 30-100 mcg/day, although much higher doses are often used for hair growth.

Vitamin B9 is also known as folate. Natural folates are found in food, and folic acid is the synthetic form used in supplements and fortified foods. Folate is very important for your immune system and energy production. Folate is involved in methylation reactions. It also produces SAM-e. It is important for healthy DNA production and has been said to be anticancerous. Severe deficiency can lead to neural tube defects in babies. Major food sources include green leafy vegetables, citrus fruit juices, and legumes. The recommended dosage is 400 mcg/day. Higher doses are often recommended if the patient has the need, such as if they have MTHFR genetic defects, as discussed in chapter 3. I use folate to help my patients who had abnormal PAP smears. Over and over I have seen repeat PAPs return normal in patients taking this nutrient.

Vitamin B12, also known as cobalamin, plays essential roles in folate metabolism and in the synthesis of the citric acid cycle intermediate succinyl-CoA, which means it helps you produce energy. It can also help to lower homocysteine. It is also used in the production of neurotransmitters. Severe deficiency in either folate or vitamin B12 can lead to megaloblastic (pernicious) anemia, which can cause fatigue, weakness, and shortness of breath. B12 is also very important for nerve health. Major food sources include meat, poultry, and fish. Vegan and vegetarians are often low in B12 and need to supplement. The recommended dosage is 400–2,000 mcg/day pending need.

Vitamin C is also known as ascorbic acid. Humans can't make ascorbic acid and must obtain vitamin C from foods. Vitamin C is important for wound healing and collagen synthesis. It helps the body absorb iron. It is also involved in the production of neurotransmitters. Deficiency can lead to bleeding gums, easy bruising, and frequent illness. Severe deficiency can lead to scurvy. Major food sources include the citrus fruits, chili peppers, and broccoli. Vitamin C also helps facilitate the absorption of iron. The recommended dosage is 1,000–5,000 mg/day. Too much can have a laxative effect.

Minerals

A **mineral** is an essential nutrient that comes from the earth. It can't be made by the body, but it is required by the body for performing functions necessary for life. Plants get minerals from soil and water. We get minerals from consuming plants and animals and from drinking water.

The five major "macrominerals" in the human body that I will briefly discuss are calcium, magnesium, phosphorus, potassium, and sodium. All of the remaining functional elements in a human body are called trace or "microminerals," as they are only needed by the body in trace amounts. They include copper, chromium, iron, iodine, manganese, zinc, and selenium.

Macrominerals

Calcium, not surprisingly, is the most abundant mineral in the body. It helps muscles produce energy. It is important for bone and teeth development. Severe deficiency can lead to muscle spasms, cramping and twitching, and osteoporosis. Major food sources include oily fish, kelp, dairy, greens, and nuts. The recommended dosage for older adults is typically 1,000-1,500 mg/day in divided doses, since your body only absorbs 500 mg of one type of calcium at a time. Some individuals should not supplement with calcium if they are prone to calcium oxylate kidney stones.

Magnesium is a cofactor for over three hundred enzymes in your body. It is also involved in the production of ATP. I often use magnesium to help relax the mind in order to sleep, and also to help the bowels to reduce constipation. It can help relax the nerves and blood vessels. It can also help to lower blood pressure and is excellent for headaches. Half of your body's magnesium is found in your bones. Most women with osteoporosis are more magnesium deficient than calcium deficient. Severe deficiency can lead to anxiety, panic attacks, depression, and muscle cramps. Major food sources include green leafy plants, meats, milk, and nuts. The recommended dosage is 400–800 mg/day. Too much of certain types of magnesium, such as oxide and citrate, can cause diarrhea. The preferred form for my patients is magnesium glycinate, although threonate has proven to be more useful for sleep. For a hundred and fifty more pages on this amazing nutrient, read *The Magnesium Miracle* by Carolyn Dean, MD, who discusses its use for even PMS and fibromyalgia.

Phosphorus is the second most abundant mineral in your body. It is mainly found in your bones. Severe deficiency can lead to anorexia and broken bones. The most common causes of unintentional deficiency are overconsumption of calcium and other antacids. Major food sources include plants, such as grains, legumes, and seeds. The recommended dosage for adults is 800 mg/day.

You have likely thought of **potassium** as an electrolyte. The term *electrolyte* refers to a substance that dissociates into ions (charged particles) in a solution, making it capable of conducting electricity (Higdon 2001). It stays in your body's cells. It is the most abundant intracellular cation, meaning it stays inside the cells. It is important for nerve transmission, blood pressure regulation, and muscle contraction. Severe imbalance can lead to an irregular heartbeat, muscle cramps, and central nervous system changes. Major food sources include bananas, potatoes, fruits, molasses, and beans. The recommended dosage is 500 mg/day. High amounts of potassium can cause diarrhea and death. Taking licorice root (glycyrrhiza) can lower potassium.

Sodium is also an electrolyte. Is it the main extracellular cation, meaning it stays outside the cells. It helps with your fluid volume and is also involved in nerve transmission. It is essential for nearly every cell in your body. High potassium intake reduces sodium. Imbalance can lead to confusion, headaches, weakness, and other neurological symptoms. A major way to increase sodium in your diet is to add Himalayan or Celtic sea salt. Olives, kelp, and pickles are also great sources. The recommended dosage varies. I find that my patients that exercise and sweat a lot need to supplement with more salt in their diets. I also often recommend a higher salt diet for my patients with adrenal fatigue symptoms and low blood pressure, which often go hand in hand. A high salt diet has helped me tremendously.

VITAMINS	MINERALS	AMINO ACIDS	ANTIOXIDANTS
Fat-soluble	*Macrominerals*	Arginine	Alpha Lipoic Acid (ALA)
Vitamin A	Calcium	Carnitine	CoezymeQ10 (CoQ10)
Vitamin D	Magnesium	Gamma Amino Butyric Acid (GABA)	Glutathione
Vitamin E	Phosphorus	Glutamine	
Vitamin K	Potassium	Glycine	
	Sodium	Histadine	
Water-soluble		Lysine	
Vitamin B1	*Microminerals*	L. Theanine	
Vitamin B2	Copper	Methionine	
Vitamin B3	Chromium	N Acetyl Cysteine (NAC)	
Vitamin B5	Iron	Phenylalanine	
Vitamin B6	Iodine	Taurine	
Vitamin B7	Manganese	Tryptophan	
Vitamin B9	Zinc	5-Hydroxytryptophan (5HTP)	
Vitamin B12	Selenium	Alanine	
Vitamin C	Silica	Aspartic Acid	
	Boron	Citrulline	
	Nickel	Cysteine	
	Molybdenum	Cystine	
		Isoleucine	

Microminerals

Copper is involved in energy production, iron metabolism, connective tissue maturation, and neurotransmission (Higdon 2001). It also helps provide the color to skin, pupils, and hair. Severe deficiency can lead to bone abnormalities, loss of muscle tone, and low white blood cells. Copper toxicity can occur primarily from environmental exposure and can cause kidney, liver, and brain damage. Major food sources include organ meats, shellfish, nuts, and seeds. The recommended dosage is 1.5–3 mg/day. The body's perfect ratio of zinc to copper is between 10 to 1 and 15 to 1. Supplementing copper should be avoided in those with Wilson's disease.

Chromium is very important for facilitating glucose transport into cells. Severe deficiency can lead to anxiety, heart disease, high blood sugar, and neuropathy. Major food sources include fruits, vegetables, meats, and grains. The recommended dosage is 50–200 mg/day. I often recommend it for my patients with insulin resistance. It has been known to reduce cravings.

Iron is a component of hemoglobin, which carries oxygen to your tissues. It is necessary for thyroid hormones and for converting tyrosine to dopamine. Severe deficiency can lead to hair loss, fatigue, paleness, shortness of breath, and weakness. Ice cravings may be a symptom of low iron. Major food sources include kelp, molasses, meat, poultry, and fish. The recommended dosage is 10 mg/day. The need is increased for pregnant women, often to 30 mg/day. Too much can be constipating. The iron I recommend for my patients should not be constipating, as it is bound to an amino acid and called an "amino acid chelated" product. Being chelated or bound to an amino acid helps the body facilitate its absorption of iron so that it doesn't bind to food in the gut and cause constipation. Vitamin C enhances its absorption. Many women become iron deficient due to heavy menstrual cycles. It is not recommended that individuals supplement with iron unless instructed by a medical provider. Iron is one mineral you can overdose on. If my patients are taking iron, I recommend checking iron and ferritin (iron storage) levels routinely.

Iodine is antibacterial. You may have seen topical iodine solutions used in health care for cleaning and sterilization purposes. Iodine is important for thyroid function, and it can help reduce painful fibrocystic breast symptoms. Severe deficiency during pregnancy can lead to irreversible mental and neurological impairment in the infant. Major food sources include milk, cheese, meat, kelp, seaweed, and iodized salt. Of note, Himalayan and Celtic sea salt are not iodized but do contain several other important trace minerals, unlike processed iodized salt. The recommended dosage is 150 mcg/day, although after testing and confirming that many of my patients are low, I recommend much higher dosages, specifically to help with thyroid hormone production. To learn more about the importance of iodine, check out the website of David Brownstein, MD at www.drbrownstein.com, or get a copy of his book, *Iodine: Why You Need It and Why You Can't Live Without It.*

Manganese is a mineral unfamiliar to many people. It is involved in producing chondroitin sulfate, which many people are more familiar with. It is important for cartilage and bone. Severe deficiency can lead to bone and joint abnormalities. Manganese toxicity has been found in miners exposed to manganese dust and can cause neurological symptoms like psychosis. Major food sources include grains, nuts, leafy vegetables, and teas. The recommended dosage is 2.5–5 mg/day. However, most individuals consume enough manganese in food and do not need to supplement.

Zinc is also a cofactor for numerous enzymes. It is essential for growth and development. Severe deficiency can lead to lack of taste, immune deficiencies, white spots on nails, and even nerve damage. It is necessary for hormone production, specifically testosterone. Major food sources include oysters, ginger root, meat, eggs, and seafood. The recommended dosage is 10 mg/day. Taking too much zinc can deplete copper.

Selenium is important for converting thyroxine (T4) into triiodothyronine (T3), as well as for producing glutathione. It is also important for several organs. Severe deficiency can lead to hair loss and growth delays. Selenium has been said to help reduce side effects of chemotherapy. Major food sources include organ meats, seafood, and Brazil nuts. Selenium is one of the minerals you can become toxic in, producing neurological symptoms like depression, convulsions, and paralysis. The recommended dosage is 55–200 mcg/day.

Other important microminerals that I won't detail here include silica, boron, nickel, and molybdenum.

AMINO ACIDS

Amino acids link proteins through peptide bonds. Amino acids make up the genetic code. As mentioned before, they are called the building blocks of life. It is important to take magnesium and B6 with nearly every amino acid to help it metabolize properly.

Our bodies can't make **essential amino acids**, so it is necessary to obtain them from food. These amino acids include histadine, isoleucine, leucine, lysine, methionine, phenylalanine, threonine, tryptophan, and valine.

Nonessential amino acids are made by your body. These include alanine, asparagine, aspartic acid, carnitine, glutamic acid, glycine, proline, and serine.

Conditionally essential amino acids are also made by your body, but may need to be ingested in times of stress, such when you have a poor diet, are ill, or your body is experiencing an infection. These include arginine, cysteine, glutamine, taurine, and tyrosine (Sahley and Birkner 2011).

The following are the amino acids I have found the most useful in my practice. I have seen patients' mental health greatly benefit from supplementing with amino acids. They assist with pain, stress, anxiety, and depression, because they ultimately help build neurotransmitters, which are the "chemical language of the brain," allowing brain cells to communicate with each other (Sahley and Birkner 2011, 12). Neurons and other brain cells have mitochondria inside them. Mitochondria are the powerhouse of the cell, providing the cell with energy. Mitochondria must be fed with vitamins, minerals, amino acids, fatty acids, and antioxidants. When well fed, they can produce the neurotransmitters your body needs.

Drugs do not increase neurotransmitters the way an amino acid can. They only inhibit the reuptake into the cell allowing more to float around, or they stimulate excessive increases of what neurotransmitter stores already exist. Drugs use up what neurotransmitters are available, but over time, if the stores are used up, the effect of the medication may go away. That is why so many individuals feel they build a tolerance to a drug, causing it to stop working. Amino acids, on the other hand, do help boost production.

The names of some amino acids have an L or D associated with them. L is Latin for "levo," or "left." D is Latin for "devo," or "right." These refer to the rotation of the structure of the molecule. Typically, proteins in plants and animals are made from "L" forms of amino acids, and they are believed to be better absorbed and more compatible for human use.

Arginine is popular among my male patients. It helps build muscle and enhances fat metabolism, and it can also help to increase growth hormone and increase sperm count and motility. It's also very important for circulation. It is essential for the production of nitric oxide (NO), and thus has been said to help reduce erectile dysfunction, Raynaud's, and high blood pressure. Severe deficiency can lead to fatty liver, hair loss and breakage, and poor wound healing. Major food sources include carob, chocolate, cabbage, dairy, meat, eggs, poultry, and raisins. The recommended dosage is 1,000–3,000 mg/day. Take caution if you have herpes. Arginine can deplete lysine, which helps with viruses. Boost your lysine by taking one gram daily for a week before you start taking arginine if you struggle with herpes.

Carnitine can increase muscle strength. It is excellent for the heart as well as for the brain. It helps transport long-chain fatty acids into cells so that fats can be used for energy production. The favorite form, acetyl-L-carnitine, helps neurons release the neurotransmitters acetylcholine and dopamine. Severe deficiency is a rare genetic disorder. Major food sources include meat, poultry, fish, and dairy products. The recommended dosage is 1,000–2,000 mg/day.

Gamma Amino Butyric Acid (GABA) is a popular soothing, calming amino. It slows down and blocks excitatory signals. It is beneficial for stress, anxiety, depression, and pain. It can be used as a natural muscle relaxant. It is excellent for sleep. Severe deficiency can lead to anxiety and racing thoughts. Major food sources include beans, eggs, nuts, and poultry. The recommended dosage is often based on weight, starting at 375 mg one to three times daily, depending on the formulation.

Glutamine was already discussed in the **Repair** section of chapter 1. Glutamine is a precursor to the calming amino acid GABA. It has been said that glutamine can enhance the effectiveness of chemotherapy and radiation while also reducing havoc on the body (Sahley and Birkner 2011).

Glycine is another calming amino acid. It is helpful for calming the nervous system and for collagen formation. It also helps detoxify heavy metals and toxins. It is necessary for making hemoglobin, glutathione, DNA, and RNA. It can be used as a sweetener, and it reduces sweet cravings. Some believe it can be helpful in reducing gout by increasing uric acid excretion. Major food sources include seaweed, spirulina, meats, and eggs. The recommended dosage is 500–3,000 mg/day.

Histadine is important for the myelin sheath that protects our nerves. Histadine is a precursor to histamine. High histamine is found in individuals with chronic pain and fibromyalgia. Major food sources include meat, pork, cheese, and wheat germ. Research suggests that reducing high-histamine foods can help reduce migraines and pain. Low-histamine diet is discussed in chapter 1.

Lysine is important for making proteins, repairing tissue, and producing hormones, and can also help reduce viral outbreaks like herpes. Lysine can also help remove heavy metals like lead from the body. Severe deficiency can lead to fatigue, anemia, poor concentration, growth delays, hair loss, and reproductive problems. Major food sources include meat, dairy, and beans. The recommended dosage varies, starting at 500 mg/day and ranging up to 3,000 mg/day short term for herpes outbreaks. Lysine antagonizes or depletes arginine.

L-theanine converts to GABA in the brain. It comes from green tea leaves. It has become a popular calming amino acid. It helps induce alpha brain waves and a relaxed state. It is helpful for sleep, anxiety, and stress. It counteracts the effects of caffeine, and can help improve focus and concentration. Severe deficiency can lead to agitation. Major food sources include green tea, although you'd have to drink four to five cups a day to equal 500 mg. The recommended dosage is 100–200 mg one to four times a day. This is one of my favorite products, and a supplement I have used often in times of stress to help calm my nerves.

Methionine is a sulfur-containing amino acid and a methyl donor, which can help to reduce elevated levels of homocysteine. It helps with detoxification and reducing fat accumulation in the liver. It is important for selenium to be absorbed by the body. It can help to reduce high histamine levels. It is important for the formation or neurotransmitters. Severe deficiency can lead to liver damage, swelling, and weakness. Major food sources include meat, fish, and grains. The recommended dosage is 800–1,000 mg/day. It has been reported to interfere with levodopa, a Parkinson's drug.

N-acetylcysteine (NAC) is a modified form of the conditionally essential amino acid cysteine. Cysteine helps build hair, fingernails, and skin. It also helps destroy nasty chemicals from drinking and smoking, such as acetaldehyde, because it helps boost glutathione levels (discussed later in this chapter). Tylenol is very hard on the liver. I recommend when my patients take it to also supplement with NAC, as NAC is also used to treat Tylenol poisoning. I also remember giving it to patients in the hospital in a medication called Mucomyst, which they inhaled. It smelled terribly like rotten eggs. NAC is a mucous-reducing agent, and is great for respiratory issues. It is used to help loosen mucus in the airways and thin the viscosity of their secretions, similar to Mucinex. It is in various allergy/respiratory products that I use in my clinic. NAC is a precursor to glutathione, the most powerful antioxidant in the body. NAC can help reduce the stress on the liver and replenish glutathione stores. It is beneficial to take vitamin C with NAC to reduce kidney stone production.

Phenylalanine (PEA) is converted to tyrosine, which then converts to L-dopa, norepinephrine, and epinephrine, your excitatory neurotransmitters, also called catecholamines or endorphins, which make you feel great. Tyrosine is important for thyroid function and possibly for helping to reduce pain. PEA helps you feel full after eating, since it helps release cholecystokinin (CCK). Severe deficiency can lead to muscle loss, confusion, depression, and weakness. Major food sources include dairy, meat, and beans. The recommended dosage is 500–3,000 mg/day. PEA should not be taken if you have phenylketonuria (PKU) or if you are on MAO-inhibiting drugs or other antidepressants.

Taurine is an inhibitory or calming amino acid and is one of the sulfur amino acids. Taurine is important for health of the gallbladder, brain, heart, and eyes. Taurine is heavily depleted when you are stressed and in pain. It is helpful for those with neurological symptoms like tics and spasms. Severe deficiency can lead to anxiety, heart arrhythmias, and seizures. Major food sources include organ meats and fish. The recommended dosage is 500–3,000 mg. It should not be taken with any salicylates, such as aspirin.

Tryptophan is a precursor to serotonin, another calming neurotransmitter. It helps you feel calm and mellow. It is a natural antidepressant. It can also help suppress appetite. Some believe it can help calm restless legs. Severe deficiency can lead to impaired growth and weight loss. Major food sources include bananas, turkey, avocados, beans, dairy, and meat. The recommended dosage is 5–50 mg/day. Many individuals opt to instead supplement with **5HTP**. Tryptophan should be avoided or used with caution if the patient is on antidepressant medications.

5-hydroxytryptophan (5HTP) is ten times stronger than tryptophan. It comes from tryptophan, then converts to serotonin and melatonin. It can help with sleep, anxiety, and depression. The recommended dosage is 50–300 mg daily. It, too, should be avoided or used with caution if the patient is on antidepressant medications.

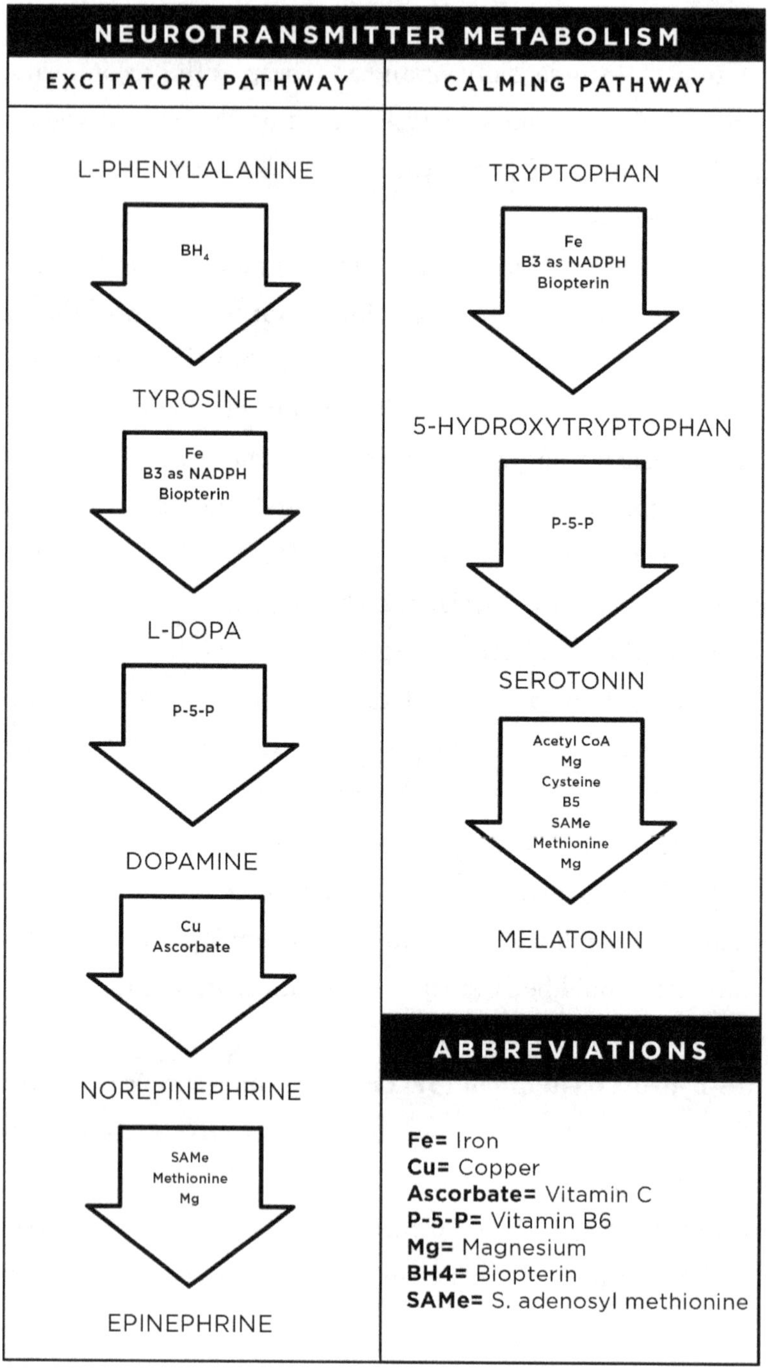
NEUROTRANSMITTER METABOLISM
EXCITATORY PATHWAY
CALMING PATHWAY
L-PHENYLALANINE
BH4
TYROSINE
Fe
B3 as NADPH
Biopterin
L-DOPA
P-5-P
DOPAMINE
Cu
Ascorbate
NOREPINEPHRINE
SAMe
Methionine
Mg
EPINEPHRINE
TRYPTOPHAN
Fe
B3 as NADPH
Biopterin
5-HYDROXYTRYPTOPHAN
P-5-P
SEROTONIN
Acetyl CoA
Mg
Cysteine
B5
SAMe
Methionine
Mg
MELATONIN
ABBREVIATIONS
Fe= Iron
Cu= Copper
Ascorbate= Vitamin C
P-5-P= Vitamin B6
Mg= Magnesium
BH4= Biopterin
SAMe= S. adenosyl methionine

Tyrosine converts to L-dopa, norepinephrine, and epinephrine—your excitatory neurotransmitters mentioned previously. It is important for building thyroid hormones. Severe deficiency can lead to low thyroid function and depression. Major food sources include dairy, meat, and beans. The recommended dosage is 500–2,000 mg/day. Monitor your blood pressure on this medication, since it can cause a rise or decrease, and do not take it if you are on an MAO-inhibiting medication.

Other important amino acids include alanine, aspartic acid, citrulline, cysteine, cystine, and isoleucine.

ESSENTIAL FATTY ACIDS

Essential fatty acids, specifically omega-3s, were introduced in the **Repair** section of chapter 1. Your brain is 60 percent fat. You need fat for your body to function. Fats are important for the neurological development of babies and children. They are needed for mental and cardiovascular health, and can even help with skin conditions like eczema and psoriasis.

Major food sources of omegas include seeds, nuts, and fish. The top source I recommend that my patients consume is fish. When you eat fish, choose small fish, which are higher in healthy oils and lower in heavy metals like mercury. Big fish eat smaller fish, which eat smaller fish, increasing the levels of metals.

People often think they need to eat fish specifically to increase their omegas, but think about it—fish eat plants. Humans can also obtain omegas from plants such as algae. Plants are a great source of fatty acids for people who are allergic to fish.

Omega-3 deficiencies can lead to a variety of symptoms, including numbness, weakness, tingling sensations, and even blurred vision (Gaby 2011). To learn more about fat, I highly encourage you to read *The Queen of Fats* by Susan Allport. High doses of fish oil can cause loose stools, diarrhea, and other gastrointestinal side effects. Omega-3s also inhibit platelet aggregation, which means your clotting is delayed. This is one benefit, but be aware that if you have a cut or scrape, pressure may need to be applied to the wound for a longer period of time. Also, if you want to take fish oil, alert your medical provider if you take aspirin, nonsteroidal anti-inflammatory drugs (NSAIDs), or coumadin.

ANTIOXIDANTS

Antioxidants help to protect your cells. They stop cell damage caused by oxidants or free radicals, which attack healthy cells. Free radicals contain an unpaired electron, so they are considered unstable and reach out to capture electrons from other substances in order to neutralize themselves. This initially stabilizes the free radical but generates another in the process, eliciting a terrible chain reaction. Having high oxidation in your body is not a good thing. It is often compared to rust on a car. It must be stopped. Daily exposure to smoke, alcohol, toxins in the air or in food, and radiation from televisions and cell phones subjects you to free radicals.

Antioxidants are found in foods like tomatoes (due to lycopene), chocolate (due to flavanols), tea, coffee, wine (containing resveratrol), fruits, and veggies. Antioxidants are said to be very antiaging, anticancerous, and immune boosting.

NAC and vitamins A, E, and C have antioxidant properties.

Alpha lipoic acid (ALA) is an antioxidant. It can help with insulin signaling and promotes the regeneration of glutathione. It has been shown to help with diabetes, diabetic neuropathies, multiple sclerosis, and can even boost glutathione. Severe deficiency can lead to neuropathies. Major food sources include meat, liver, spinach, and broccoli. The recommended dosage is 300–1,200 mg/day.

Coezyme Q10 (CoQ10) is also known as ubiquinone. The active form is ubiquinol, which is better absorbed by the body. As we age, converting ubiquinone to ubiquinol becomes less efficient. Those over fifty-five I recommend taking ubiquinol. It is a fat-soluble antioxidant, and it is depleted by various blood pressure and cholesterol-lowering medications. It is necessary for the mitochondrial production of adenosine triphosphate (ATP), an energy source converter. It can also help with fatigue and is most popular for its help with cardiovascular diseases like heart failure and high blood pressure. It can prevent your cholesterol from oxidation. It also protects cells from death. I've found it helps reduce headaches in my patients. Severe deficiency can lead to cardiovascular complications like heart failure. Major food sources include meat, poultry, fish, beans, and eggs. The recommended dosage is 30–300 mg/day.

Glutathione, as mentioned, is the most powerful antioxidant in the body, which protects you from free radical damage. It literally protects your DNA. It is helpful for DNA repair. It is made of three amino acids, cysteine, glutamic acid, and glycine. Glutathione is extremely important to the liver for helping with detoxification. It helps you get rid of toxins like heavy metals. Taking Tylenol, smoking, and drinking alcohol will deplete your glutathione levels. Suzy Cohen, author of *Drug Muggers*, says, "You pretty much use up all your glutathione just for eating, never mind dealing with drug muggers and lifestyle choices" (Cohen 2011, 143). Severe deficiency can lead to fatigue and autoimmune conditions and cancer. Major food sources include asparagus, avocado, garlic, green veggies, and beets. The recommended dosage is 1,000–3,000 mg/day.

WHY ARE WE NUTRITIONALLY DEFICIENT?

No one wants to be deficient on any of the aforementioned nutrients, especially when it's so simple to fix the deficiencies. Having even subtle deficiencies won't allow your body to unlock necessary doors. That's a simple way of saying these deficiencies can lead to DNA damage, which then leads to chronic disease and cancer.

Why are we so nutritionally deficient? With age, people make less of many nutrients, and their digestive processes start to decline, but that's not all. There are several other reasons.

Remember Jared, from earlier in this chapter? Jared ate terribly. He, like possibly many of you reading this book, ate the typical Standard American Diet (SAD). He essentially knew he was setting himself up for nutritional deficiencies. Fast food is processed and doesn't contain the nutrients and enzymes that fresh food does. Karen was aging and was taking omeprazole. As mentioned in chapter 1, without a healthy foundation and healthy digestion, you unfortunately won't be reaping all the benefits from the food you ingest. If your digestion or absorption is poor, you can be left nutritionally deficient. That's why the gut is the foundation of your Longevity Blueprint. Many of my patients continue to wonder why they can't receive all the nutrition they need from food just as their grandparents did. Times have changed. Let's learn why.

WAYS FOOD LOSES NUTRIENTS	
Deficient soil	Storing
Harvesting	Freezing
Processing	Cooking with high heat

Deficient Soil

Since the 1950s, the nutrient content in our foods has been on the decline. US Department of Agriculture (USDA) figures demonstrate a decline in over forty crops that the agency tracks (USDA). For instance, it has been estimated that magnesium content in foods has declined 25 to 80 percent (Ancient Minerals 2015). Why? Sources suggest that this is for several reasons, two of which are over-farmed, depleted soils, and the processing of foods (Ancient Minerals 2015). Let me be clear, we need farmers. Being from Nebraska, and living in Iowa now, half of my family farms. However, farming has changed. Farmers used to use manure for fertilizing, and now they use pesticides and chemical fertilizers. They used to rotate crops more than they do now, which helped to suppress insects and diseases.

Our foods are the product of our **soil**. I think we often forget that. If the soil has been robbed of magnesium, would we expect our food to be any different? Soil should be rich in antioxidants, vitamins, and minerals, producing foods high in the same.

As I mentioned earlier, vegetarians should supplement with B12, since their vegetable-based diet is low in B12. But did you know that this didn't use to be true? Root vegetables used to be higher in B12. Because of the use of pesticides and herbicides ridding the ground of living weeds, earthworms, and natural fertilizers, the soil has been dramatically altered. Extinguishing the ground from this living vegetation is primarily why the vitamin and mineral content has declined.

The herbicide atrazine is cheap and popular. It can be applied to crops to control weeds before they emerge. But did you know that it can cause mitrochondrial dysfunction, which is the term for ridding the body of the ability to create energy? It can also cause insulin resistance and diabetes.

I always wondered how farmers get rid of remaining herbicides and pesticides after they've covered their land. Or what about accidental spills? I've read of farmers dumping the remains into nearby ditches or streams. This is obviously going back into our water system. Overgrazing and not rotating crops leads to increased dependence on pesticides. And if you think those herbicides and pesticides aren't getting into our water, you are crazy! We used to fish in a little pond on my grandpa's farmland. At the time, I wasn't thinking about the fact that the fish I was so proud to catch and eat likely had been contaminated with herbicides and pesticides that had run down from the farmland.

In *Silent Spring*, author Rachel Carson discusses how hazardous these chemicals are to animals (Carson 1962). Dichlorodiphenyltrichloroethane (DDT), for instance, was found to have accumulated in fish, reptiles, birds, and mammals (Carson 1962). Yet we assume we won't be affected. Wrong! Insecticides can kill birds and fish. They are likely more harmful to humans than herbicides, because we are more similar to insects than we are to plants. Herbicides can damage our DNA. They certainly kill earthworms. I had no idea how valuable those little free workers were until I attended a conference where our devastating soil loss was discussed. Worms help preserve and save our soil, because their burrows soak up water from rain, which would otherwise erode the soil.

Again, all these chemicals destroy the natural biological activity and deplete the soil of necessary nutrients, resulting in nutrient-deficient foods. Living near factories (which manufacture high fructose corn syrup, I must add), I can see the pollution chugging into the air daily, and often I can smell it. That pollution essentially comes right back down on our farmlands in the form of contaminated rains.

No doubt, industrialization has contributed to our lands and waters becoming contaminated.

Processing

It was already known back in the 1930s that processing foods depletes their nutrients (like vitamins and minerals). Processed foods were created in war time so that we could ship food long distances. The best way to prevent food from going bad is to remove the nutrients that attract bacteria and insects. When food is processed, ingredients that "go bad" are removed. Real food "goes bad," because it is truly alive. These things that "go bad" are what you should be eating. You should choose to eat *only* foods that will eventually go bad or rot—foods that fungi and bacteria actually want.

Food processing separates plant food sources, often removing the portion containing most of the nutrients, such as magnesium. For example, a safflower seed contains 680 mg magnesium per 100 calories, yet when the seed is processed into refined oil, the final product contains no magnesium (Seelig and Rosanoff 2003).

Our foods are also mostly of the same variety, the high-performing variety. So we buy one type of chicken, one type of broccoli, and one type of corn. Also, it's been said that 75 percent of the vegetable oils we now consume are from either corn or soy (Pollan 2007). Because we can extract carbs from corn and fats and protein from soy, we can now find corn and soy in the majority of processed foods in our grocery stores.

Harvesting/Picking

Foods also start to lose their nutritional value once they are picked. The average time between when a food is harvested and when it is eaten varies. It's been said that produce loses 30–90 percent of its nutrients in the three days after harvest (Eng 2013). It would be ideal to have your own garden and pick your food immediately before dinner. That would preserve the most nutritional value possible.

Storing and Cooking at High Temps

Storing processes like canning and freezing can also reduce nutritional value in foods, although the results of studies are variable. Cooking at high temperatures for long periods of time can also reduce nutrient content in food, since it can cause proteins to denature or come apart. B vitamins and vitamin C are water soluble, and, when cooked with water, these vitamins can leach out of the food into the water. Microwave cooking can also be dangerous, due to the radiation and the container you are cooking your food in. For instance, cooking plastic under that high heat can cause dangerous toxins to leach into your foods. If you use a microwave, use a safe container like glass.

Medications

Were you vaccinated as a child and have you taken any medications? I could write an entire chapter on how medications cause nutrient deficiencies. Shoot, Suzy Cohen, who is known as "America's Most Trusted Pharmacist," wrote an entire 371 page book on it! In *Drug Muggers*, she discusses how we take medications hoping they will make us feel better, yet we often end up feeling sicker (Cohen 2011). She understands that medications are needed to help reduce pain or help you breathe, for instance, but she also understands that drugs don't cure anything (Cohen 2011). They simply help reduce symptoms. If we ate healthier, we likely wouldn't need as many nutrients or the drugs for our symptoms. Pollen says it best, "Medicine is learning how to keep alive the people whom the Western diet is making sick" (Pollen 2008, 135).

Cohen's whole book is about helping the patient stay safe on the medications they take. She coined the term "drug mugger," which she defines as "an over-the-counter (OTC) or prescribed medication, food, herb, medical condition, or lifestyle choice that is capable of robbing your body's natural stores of an important vitamin, mineral or hormone" (Cohen 2011, 7).

And this "mugging" or depletion doesn't just happen the day you take a drug—it can happen for weeks to months afterward. If you have high blood pressure, you have it for a reason, not because you lack blood pressure medication in your body. Unfortunately, when you take the blood pressure medication, you now lack other nutrients it has "mugged" you of. It is essential we replenish the nutrients that drugs steal from our bodies.

To review the drugs you take and the nutrients they deplete, check out Cohen's very thorough book with her "nutrient security system." She has a list of common drug muggers. Here are a few of special note:

- **Statin drugs** for cholesterol, **blood pressure reducing** and **diabetic drugs** deplete the body of CoQ10.
- **Diabetic drugs** (such as metformin)**, antibiotics,** and **heartburn drugs** (such as omeprazole or cimetidine) deplete the body of B vitamins, such as B12.
- **Blood pressure medications**, **heartburn drugs**, **antibiotics**, and **inhaled steroids** deplete the body of magnesium.
- **Diuretics** make you urinate, depleting essential nutrients.
- **Birth control medications** deplete the body of B vitamins and magnesium.

- **Antidepressants** rob the body of B vitamins as well. If you are depressed, it's likely that you are already low on nutrients, since they are essential for making neurotransmitters like serotonin. If you are then placed on an antidepressant, it further robs you of the vital nutrients you needed more of to begin with!
- **Thyroid medications** can deplete you of calcium and iron.
- **Laxatives** essentially make food go through you more quickly, so your body doesn't have time for proper absorption.
- **Antacids and acid blockers** reduce acid, which is necessary for proper absorption. Long-term use of laxatives almost guarantees deficiencies.
- **Antibiotics** kill off good bacteria, allowing yeast to overgrow, which can also interfere with the absorption of nutrients.

Do you want to know more? Great resources for nutrient deficiencies caused by medications can be found on the SpectraCell Laboratories website at www.spectracell.com.

BRAND NAME EXAMPLES	NUTRIENTS DEPLETED
ANTACIDS	
Pepcid, Tagamet, Zantac	Vitamin B12, Folate, Vitamin D, Calcium, Iron, Zinc
Prevacid, Prilosec	Vitamin B12
ANTIBIOTICS	
General Aminoglycosides (gentomycin, neomycin, streptomycin), Cephalosporins, Penicillins	B vitamins, Vitamin K, Friendly Beneficial Intestinal Bacteria
Tetracycllines	Calcium, Zinc, Magnesium, Iron, Vitamin B6
ANTI-DIABETIC DRUGS	
Micronase, Tolinase	Coenzyme Q10
Glucophage	Coenzyme Q10, Vitamin B12, Folate
ANTIDEPRESSANTS	
Adapin, Aventyl, Elavil, Tofranil, Pamelor, Sinequan, Norpramin	Vitamin B12, Coenzyme Q10
ANTI-INFLAMMATORIES	
Aspirin & Salicylates	Vitamin C, Folate, Iron, Potassium,
Advil, Aleve, Anaprox, Dolobid, Feldene, Lodine, Motrin, Naprosyn, Orudis, Relafen	Folate
Betamethasone, Cortisone, Dexamethasone, Hydrocortisone, Methylprednisolone, Prednisone	Vitamin C, Vitamin D, Folate, Calcium, Magnesium, Potassium, Selenium, Zinc
CARDIOVASCULAR DRUGS	
Apresoline	Vitamin B6, Coenzyme Q10
Catapres, Aldomet	Coenzyme Q10
DIURETICS	
Lasix, Bumex, Edecrin	Vitamin B1, Vitamin B6, Vitamin C, Magnesium, Calcium, Potassium, Zinc, Sodium
Enduron, Diuril, Lozol, Zaroxolyn, Hygroton	Magnesium, Potassium, Zinc, Coenzyme Q10, Sodium

BRAND NAME EXAMPLES	NUTRIENTS DEPLETED
CHOLESTEROL LOWERING AGENTS (STATINS)	
Lescol, Lipitor, Mevacor, Zocor, Pravachol, Crestor	Coenzyme Q10
Colestid, Questran	Vitamin A, Vitamin B12, Vitamin D, Vitamin E, Vitamin K, Beta-Carotene, Folate, Iron
ULCER MEDICATIONS	
Tagamet, Pepcid, Zantac	Vitamin B12, Vitamin D, Folate, Calcium, Iron, Zinc, Protein
Prevacid, Prilosec	Vitamin B12, Protein
HRT—HORMONE REPLACEMENT THERAPY	
Evista, Prempro, Premarin, Estratab	Vitamin B2, Vitamin B6, Vitamin B12, Vitamin C, Folate, Magnesium, Zinc
ORAL CONTRACEPTIVES	
Norinyl, Ortho-Novum, Triphasil, etc.	Vitamin B2, Vitamin B3, Vitamin B6, Vitamin B12, Vitamin C, Folate, Magnesium, Selenium, Zinc

Lifestyle Toxins

In general, we live in a toxic world. Exposure to toxins requires higher nutrient levels to rid our body of these toxins (more on detoxing in the next chapter).

Think of the artificial colors, flavors, and sweeteners in our foods. These are all toxins. They are difficult for our body to deal with. Personal care products also contain toxins that can tax the liver.

Alcohol and caffeine (coffee and non-herbal tea) also rob your body of nutrients. When you drink alcohol, it is metabolized or converted to acetaldehyde, which is highly toxic to your brain—that's what causes a hangover. Coffee and teas contain tannins, which can leach minerals from your body. It's no secret that caffeine has a diuretic effect. In addition, metabolizing these three all require nutrients. This means that when you drink alcohol, coffee, and non-herbal tea, you are increasing your need to supplement.

What about soda pop? Soda pop is highly acidic and high in phosphoric acid, which also leaches minerals like calcium from your bones to help neutralize or buffer the acidic pH. It is also high in other toxins, such as sugar, that depletes your body of minerals, and often high in high fructose corn syrup. The artificial sweeteners in most sodas contain excitotoxins, which damage your cells until they burn out and die.

Do you smoke? Toxins from cigarettes and marijuana deplete you of vitamin C. I see high levels of cadmium in many of my patients who aren't even currently smoking, but who have a history of smoking. Have you ever taken OTC fat blockers for weight loss? These block your absorption of fats, even healthy fats. Exercising requires more nutrients. The harder you work out, the more nutrients your body uses up, and thus the more you need to obtain from food or supplements.

Further deficiencies can exist based on your diet if you are vegan or vegetarian. Even the area where you live in the United States can result in deficiencies. If you are pregnant, nursing, or elderly, your needs also increase. So, how do you truly know if you are low in nutrients? A functional medicine provider should be able to perform a physical exam and gather history and data suggesting what you need. However, the best way to know is to test!

TESTING FOR NUTRITIONAL DEFICIENCIES

Vitamin levels can be tested in the blood, and metabolites (organic acids) can be tested in the urine. It's important to assess one's genetics as well (see chapter 3), since many individuals will inherit genetic variants associated with nutrient deficiencies.

The most common test I run in my patients specifically looking for nutritional deficiencies is called a NutraEval through Genova Diagnostics. It's a twenty-page nutritional analysis looking at vitamins, minerals, amino acids, antioxidants, and even omega levels. It's truly amazing what insights this test can provide.

As a functional medicine provider I can often guess what nutrients a patient needs, but having confirmation from testing is very helpful. For instance, I may suspect a patient has low potassium with leg cramps, yet upon testing discover that she needs more magnesium. Additionally, testing vitamin D levels helps provide insight into just how high a dose a patient needs. I *still* have patients whose primary care providers only recommend a dose of 1,000 IU D3 for a deficient state. That's not going to budge them a single point. These individuals need high doses, which is safest to give after confirming the need through testing.

It's also truly amazing how many patients of mine *know* they feel better when their nutritional needs are met. The nutritional test has pages of data. Often, once some of my more informed patients have seen how high their need is for certain nutrients, they'll ask if their digestion and absorption is optimal. I love it when they think like that. They are trying to get to the root cause of their problem.

Interestingly, the nutritional test also contains some bacterial and yeast dysbiosis markers—which, if high, suggest we should pursue a comprehensive stool test looking for pathogens contributing to gut inflammation and poor digestion and absorption. I've had several patients with dry eyes benefit from taking higher doses of fish oil, as well as patients with brittle, thinning hair and nails benefit from amino acids and biotin, and patients who have lost their taste or smell due to eating disorders gain these senses back simply by taking zinc, which fixes their nutritional deficiencies.

ADMINISTERING THE FIX FOR NUTRITIONAL DEFICIENCIES

There are several easy ways to fix nutritional deficiencies. Various routes of administration exist, and I always discuss this with my patients, because I want them to be compliant and take what I recommend. **Oral delivery** simply means taken by mouth. Unfortunately, oral dosing can't provide 100 percent absorption, but it is the most common way my patients take their nutrients. I prefer capsules over tablets. Liquids and powders are also acceptable.

Some patients don't like swallowing pills—period. Maybe they easily choke and would prefer a liquid over a capsule. Maybe they are on acid blockers and get easily nauseated with tablets. There are several reasons I might instead suggest a **sublingual (SL) pill** that stays under the tongue for a few minutes until it dissolves, or until it is easily chewed before swallowing. These SL options and are absorbed through the mucous membranes in the mouth. The advantage with these is that the supplement bypasses the gut entirely and gets directly into the bloodstream.

Beyond oral delivery, **intravenous (IV) nutrition**—where nutrients are received directly into the bloodstream through an IV—is becoming more popular. One of the reasons why is because low stomach acid also inhibits proper absorption of nutrients taken by mouth. IV is the best delivery method, as it brings the nutrients right into the bloodstream, entirely bypassing digestion. IV therapy overcomes any current digestion or absorption issues with the patient, including the food sensitivities mentioned in chapter 1.

Research shows that administering nutrients intravenously can raise blood levels higher than when given in oral or SL form. Intravenous vitamin C can be used as an adjunct in treating cancer and supporting the immune system to fight acute and chronic infections. Vitamin C can also help support the adrenal glands. A "Myer's cocktail" contains B1, B5, B6, calcium, B9, magnesium, and vitamin C. It is excellent for chronic fatigue, fibromyalgia, and mood enhancement. Obviously, risks can be higher with IV administration. These include bruising or redness at the IV site if it becomes blocked (infiltrates). Also, serious reactions include dropping of blood pressure or heart rate and anaphylaxis. If you are interested in receiving IV vitamins, I recommend you work only with a licensed clinician who, like me, is certified in providing IV nutrients.

HOW TO SELECT HIGH QUALITY PRODUCTS

Now that I've made a case for supplementation, you probably want know where to find the best products. I've heard many analogies comparing your body to a car. If you had a Porsche, would you put cheap gas in it? Of course not! Similarly, when you purchase nutrients for your body, the most amazing machinery you possess, you need to fuel it with the highest quality gas (nutrients). It has been reported that over 60 percent of Americans take dietary supplements, and that those who do so live longer (Council for Responsible Nutrition 2015). This may be due to the fact that these individuals have invested more in their health in general. Nevertheless, working to replenish your low nutrients is not harmful, but helpful. So here are some tips for purchasing high quality products.

Read labels. Read the label to better understand exactly what you are taking. For instance, when selecting an omega-3 product, I typically recommend patients look for products from small fish. Don't take fish oil from tuna or salmon, as those are big fish with more mercury. Look at the label to see if the fish oil is sourced from sardines and anchovies, which are smaller. Also make sure the product is refined and distilled to remove any heavy metals. Research the company to verify that the fish weren't captured in contaminated water. Also make sure the product has a decent amount of EPA/DHA in it. Some omega-3 product labels make the claim on the front to contain "1,000 mg omega-3s," but when you read the label on the back, they may only have 120 mg EPA and 230 mg DHA. That's not 1,000 mg. A filler with no therapeutic value may be making up the remaining 650 mg there. As mentioned in chapter 1, I recommend many of my patients take higher doses of omega-3s—near 3,000 mg, with combined EPA and DHA. Not everyone needs that high of a dose. Get your omega-3 index checked to know for sure. It's a part of the nutritional evaluation I like to order on every patient. Another example: know the source when purchasing calcium. Cheap calcium is like eating chalk from a chalkboard. Gross! Some calcium products, like Tums, even contain heavy metals. It's no secret—you can read it right on the label. Heavy metals are something you definitely want to avoid.

The label will also reveal whether your supplements are gluten-free, and whether it's free of any other ingredients that your body is sensitive or allergic to. That includes the capsule itself along with any nasty additives that might be contained within, such as artificial colors, flavors, and sweeteners. One popular fiber supplement on the market contains aspartame. That doesn't make sense to me, since many patients who need fiber have irritable bowel syndrome and likely can't tolerate aspartame. Also avoid fillers and preservatives; they are simply unnecessary. You don't need parabens in your vitamins.

"One-a-day" multivitamin is "not the way." There's no way any company can put high doses of nutrients into one tiny pill. If they try to heat up all those nutrients and compress them all into that tablet, chances are the nutrients become destroyed. The recommended dose of most high-quality multivitamins is four to six capsules a day—*not* one a day.

In general, avoid tablets. To demonstrate why, drop both a tablet and a capsule into a cup of water—the capsule will dissolve first. Capsules are easier for your body to break down, especially if you have low stomach acid. As I mentioned earlier, I approve of liquids and powders, too. However, speaking in terms of digestion, the contents of a delayed-release capsule will make if farther down into your system, allowing for better absorption than a liquid or powder would. Again, the sublingual (SL) under-the-tongue delivery system is also excellent, allowing nutrients to go right into your blood system. In short, **choose the best absorbed version of the nutrient**. For instance, take pyridoxal 5'-phosphate (P5P) instead of B6, take methylcobalamin instead of cyanocobalamin, and take folate instead of folic acid.

Reputation matters. Most brands that are available from a licensed clinician are high quality. Think about it: in recommending that brand, the clinician is putting his or her name and reputation on the line. If they've done the necessary research, they should really only be offering what they feel is the best for you—their patient. At my practice, I've carried several brands over the years from amazing companies that test their products for purity, safety, and potency between batches and at the end of production. That's how we can, for instance, guarantee the potency of our Longevity Blueprint probiotics at the day of expiration, where many companies only do so at the day of manufacturing. So, in my clinic, if the label says it contains 20 billion CFUs, that potency is not referring to the day of manufacture—it's referring to the day of expiration, setting our brand apart. A magnesium capsule is also guaranteed to have the dose on the label at the day of expiration.

Additionally, the United States Pharmacopeia (USP) has set standards or guidelines for thc good manufacturing practice (GMP) of products. Make sure that you are purchasing supplements from somewhere that is operating up to this standard. Ask your functional medicine provider to help identify what nutrients you should be taking.

Have realistic expectations. When it comes to cost, be realistic about what you expect to pay for high quality supplements. Many high-potency probiotics cost $1 per day. If you are purchasing one that is $10 for an entire month's supply, you must question what level of quality you are getting. Don't waste a little money on junk. That goes for your lifestyle choices as well—don't spend your money on fast food and then complain that you have to supplement. Make better choices with your lifestyle, and spend your hard-earned dollar on quality supplements for your health. That's your best investment.

HOW TO SELECT **HIGH-QUALITY PRODUCTS**

1. READ LABELS
2. ONE A DAY IS NOT THE WAY
3. AVOID TABLETS
4. CHOOSE THE ACTIVE FORMS
5. CHOOSE A REPUTABLE COMPANY
6. HAVE REALISTIC EXPECTATIONS

CONCLUSION

I hope by now you are starting to feel empowered about the functional medicine options available to you.

Remember Karen and Jared? Karen learned to accept that as she aged she simply would have greater need for some nutrients. Her tests showed she needed more vitamin D and magnesium for her bones, and she also had an unexpectedly higher need for antioxidants. She was switched from salmon oil to a more potent and pure fish oil. Her food sensitivity test results were encouraging, because they helped her determine the root cause of her heartburn so that she could eventually get off her omeprazole. Jared, meanwhile, was low on nearly every nutrient because his diet was so poor. To help turn him around, I recommended he start by taking a high-quality multivitamin along with antioxidants, vitamin D, CoQ10, fish oil, and a B complex. He wasn't particularly fond of taking supplements, but doing so encouraged him to change his diet. And he began learning other ways to reduce his health risks. For instance, he started cooking fish twice a week, and reduced the number of nights he ate out each week. He also wanted to pursue additional cardiovascular testing, which I'll discuss in chapter 7.

Karen and Jared both recognized the importance of purchasing high-quality products that were well absorbed. Unlike the results Karen and Jared achieved, I've seen several repeat nutritional tests with other patients show no improvement because they wasted their money on cheap supplements that served no purpose. But with the help of a trained and experienced functional medicine provider such as myself to provide testing and high-quality products, you can identify and fix nutrient deficiencies. You can follow a Longevity Blueprint to better health.

LB carries a top-quality line of nutraceutical products and supplements. View the full line on our website, www.yourlongevityblueprint.com.

Longevity Blueprint Nutraceutical Products

Here are my favorite Longevity Blueprint nutrients.

- Mitochondrial Complex
- Complete Multi
- Complete Multi + Iron
- Magnesium Chelate
- Magnesium + Potassium Chelate
- Iron Chelate
- Calcium + Magnesium Chelate
- Zinc Chelate
- Iodine 3
- Vitamin D3 1000
- Vitamin D3 5000
- Vitamin D 5000 +K2
- Liquid D3
- Liquid D3 + K2
- Lysine
- Carnitine
- 5HTP
- Omega-3s
- Methyl B Complex
- SL Methyl Bs

- NAC
- CoQ10 100
- CoQ10 300

Chapter 4 Resources

Linus Pauling Institute: http://lpi.oregonstate.edu/

SpectraCell Laboratories: www.spectracell.com

The Queen of Fats, Susan Allport

The Magnesium Miracle, Carolyn Dean

Iodine: Why You Need It and Why You Can't Live Without It, David Brownsein

Chapter 4 References

1. Ancient Minerals. "The Bad News about Magnesium Food Sources." ancient-minerals.com (2015). http://www.ancient-minerals.com/magnesium-sources/dietary/.
2. Carson, Rachel. *Silent Spring*. New York: First Mariner Books, 2002.
3. Cohen, Suzy. *Drug Muggers*. New York: Rodale Books, 2011.
4. Eng, Monica. "Most produce loses 30 percent of nutrients three days after harvest." Chicago Tribune (July 2013). http://articles.chicagotribune.com/2013-07-10/features/chi-most-produce-loses-30-percent-of-nutrients-three-days-after-harvest-20130710_1_harvest-farmers-vitamin-c.
5. Fletcher, R.H., and K.M. Fairfield. "Vitamins for chronic disease prevention in adults: clinical applications." *The Journal of the American Medical Association* 23, no. 287 (2002). https://www.ncbi.nlm.nih.gov/pubmed/12069676.
6. Gaby, Alan. *Nutritional Medicine*. Concord, New Hampshire: Fritz Perlberg Publishing, 2011.

7. Glantz, James. *Saving Our Soil: Solutions for Sustaining Earth's Vital Resource*. Boulder, Colorado: Johnson Publishing, 1995.

8. Higdon, Jane. "Vitamin D." Linus Pauling Institute. lpi.oregonstate.edu (2000). http://lpi.oregonstate.edu/mic/vitamins/vitamin-D."

9. Higdon, Jane. "Potassium." Linus Pauling Institute. lpi.oregonstate.edu (2001). http://lpi.oregonstate.edu/mic/minerals/potassium.

10. Higdon, Jane. "Copper." Linus Pauling Institute. lpi.oregonstate.edu (2001). http://lpi.oregonstate.edu/mic/minerals/copper.

11. Pollan, Michael. *Food Rules, an Eater's Manual.* New York: Penguin Group, 2009.

12. Pollan, Michael. *In Defense of Food: An Eater's Manifesto*. London: Penguin Press, 2007.

13. Sahley, B., and K. Birkner. *Heal with Amino Acids and Nutrients*. San Antonio, Texas: Pain & Stress Publishers, 2011.

14. Seelig, M., and Rosanoff, A. *The Magnesium Factor*. New York, Avery, 2003.

15. Smith, Pam. *What You Must Know About Vitamins, Minerals, Herbs, and More: Choosing the Nutrients That Are Right for You*. Garden City Park, New York: Square One Publishers, 2008.

16. The Council for Responsible Nutrition. "The Dietary Supplement Consumer 2015 CRB Consumer Survey on Dietary Supplements." crnusa.org (2015). http://www.crnusa.org/CRNconsumersurvey/2015/.

17. Tompkins, Peter, and Christopher Bird. *Secrets of the Soil.* Anchorage, Alaska: Earthpulse Press Incorporated, 1998.

18. Wahls, T. *The Wahls Protocol: A Radical New Way to Treat All Chronic Autoimmune Conditions Using Paleo Principles.* New York: Avery, 2014.

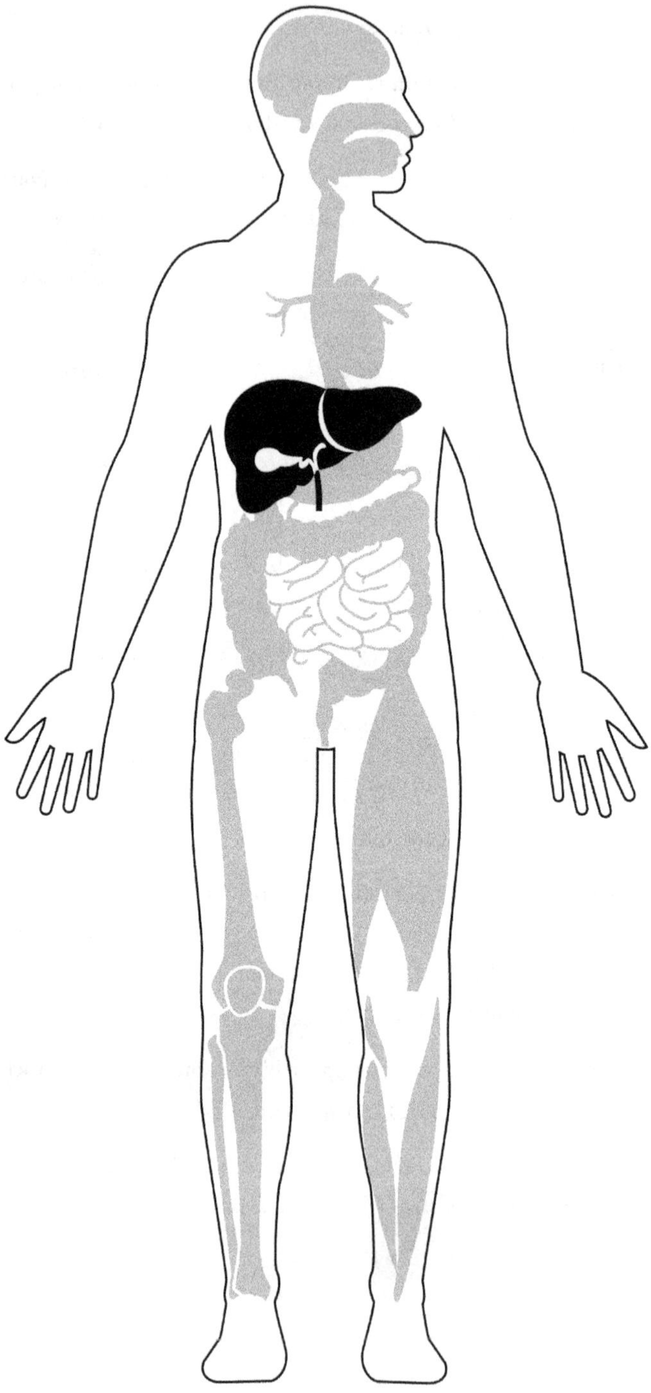

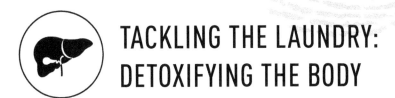

CHAPTER 5

TACKLING THE LAUNDRY: DETOXIFYING THE BODY

By cleansing your body on a regular basis and eliminating as many toxins as possible from your environment, your body can begin to heal itself, prevent disease, and become stronger and more resilient than you ever dreamed possible!

—Dr. Edward Group III

When you invite company over to your home, you want your home to look and smell good, right? Chances are, you don't want your company to see piles of smelly, dirty clothes. You want to stay caught up on the laundry. The laundry room is where there's typically a constant influx of dirty clothes that need to be cleaned, folded, and put away to be used again, only to restart this constant cycle. You can't do the laundry unless you have a functioning washing machine, water, and soap. You also likely recognize that you can't get your clothes 100 percent clean if you stuff the washing machine too full.

Some loads need to operate on gentle while other loads need the heavy-duty cycle.

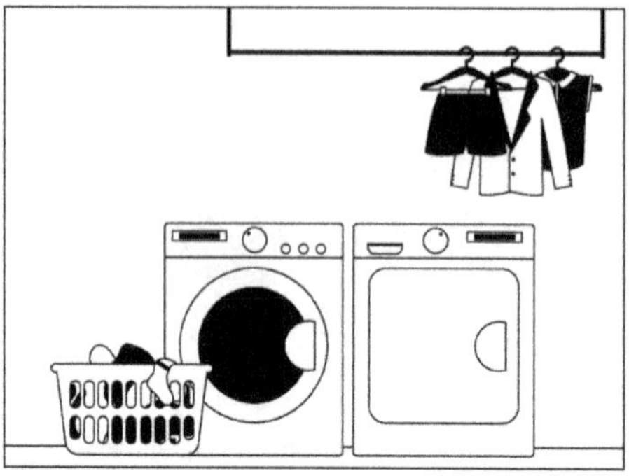

The same is true with your body. You can't powerfully detox without the essential nutrients necessary for detoxification. Your body is constantly detoxing, but sometimes the process needs to be cranked up a notch. You also need to reduce your incoming burden of toxins.

Think of this process in terms of a glass of water. If you continuously fill that glass up with water, eventually the glass can hold no more and the water will overflow. In order to fill it up again, you need to first dump out its contents. If that glass is an example of your liver and the water is the toxins it filters, imagine the load on it if it overfills. Your liver must be able to dump past toxins to prepare for the incoming new burden. That's when individuals run into trouble—when their body's toxic burden exceeds its natural ability to remove the waste.

I want to be clear on one point here. I *never* start patients on an aggressive detox program until they have worked through the first few steps of the Longevity Blueprint. The first step is to help them start to build a truly healthy foundation and work to reduce intestinal permeability or "leaky gut." If they have leaky gut and we provoke the liver to dump toxins into the gut, those toxins we are trying to get rid of will only recirculate right back into the bloodstream. The same will happen if the patient is constipated.

That's why establishing gut health is the foundation. Toxins are cleared via stool. Patients need to have regular bowel movements to detox safely. Also, patients won't detox well if they have nutritional deficiencies. These must also be fixed ahead of time. If patients purchase a "detox kit" off the internet and try to detox on their own without guidance, without following these outlined steps, they'll often end up feeling sicker quicker. I also have patients who are so toxic that they have sensitivities to everything—every food, every smell, and every supplement. These patients need to be detoxed rather gently. We must first successfully complete the first few steps in the Longevity Blueprint for these patients to successfully tolerate a gentle detox.

I have worked with some unique patients through my years in functional medicine who have shown varying levels of compliance or commitment to treatment. When treatment success isn't where it should be, the commitment of the patient is always in question, as detox is a new concept to many and can be difficult.

However, compliance wasn't the issue with one toxic young man, Scott. He was desperate for help—in fact, he had already completed a lot of research on his own. We worked him through the first few steps of the Longevity Blueprint. He strictly avoided all the foods he reacted to, but he had a GI infection (SIBO) that kept returning after treatment. He was working to reduce his stress. His hormones were balanced and nutritional deficiencies fixed. He received chiropractic adjustments every two weeks. Still, he had multiple chemical sensitivities and he felt very emotional—he complained about anxiety and sleep disturbances, and that he felt fragile for his age, having to watch everything he was exposed to and what he put in his mouth.

Although he was improving, his progress wasn't quite up to par. Finally, I told him that my instinct was that he was toxic. He was a car mechanic, and I feared his daily environmental exposure was burdening his body. His healthy lifestyle was simply not enough to keep him healthy. I agree with Debra Dadd, who stated in her book, *Toxic Free*, "Your detoxification system determines whether or not your body is sick or well" (Dadd 2011, 142).

> **"Your detoxification system determines whether or not your body is sick or well."**
> **—Debra Dadd**

Today, even chiropractors are incorporating nutrition into their practices, because they realize a simple adjustment is no longer enough to help patients with all their needs. That's because of the huge toxic load or burden that everyone carries. That was the case with Scott.

WHAT ARE TOXINS AND HOW ARE WE EXPOSED?

Toxins are any substances that have a negative effect on the human body. When toxins are in excess of the body's capacity to remove them, they store in fat until removed, because they are fat-soluble (attracted to fat). Remember, your brain is largely made of fat. You certainly don't want toxins hiding there. Yet your body and your brain are exposed to toxins everywhere—in the air you breathe, the water you drink, the foods you eat, and the chemicals you work with, whether from a computer, your cell phone, or the personal care products you use every day. For some, the home you live in could be the biggest toxic exposure.

Here are some of the toxins that we, as humans, are commonly exposed to:

Genetically Modified Organisms (GMOs) in Food

The constant exposure to various toxins happens on a daily basis, starting with what a person puts in their mouth. The average human eats nearly fifty tons of food throughout their lifetime. Now, you probably do research on vehicle safety before you purchase a family car, right? Do you put that same amount of thought into the foods you buy for your family? In the food you eat? You should. It has been estimated that the majority of the food in grocery stores is genetically modified. Many individuals think of GMOs as toxins because of the burden they put on the body. The top GMO foods include corn, soy, cottonseed, canola, and potatoes. Even if you aren't eating corn, corn derivatives like corn syrup are found in items ranging from candies to ketchup. Legislation may be in the works for better labeling, but at this point our food isn't labeled as containing GMOs. Certainly when you eat out, unless you visit a local establishment that serves organic food, you are likely getting bombarded with GMOs as well.

Why do GMOs exist? Here's an example: In a growing field, potatoes are susceptible to insects. By adding a certain gene to a potato, that potato can create its own insecticide to keep insects away. In theory, the technology sounds great, but there is no evidence yet of how gene alteration affects human bodies. Even the US Centers for Disease Control (CDC) admits that food is responsible for twice the number of illnesses in the United States as scientists thought years ago. Is that because food on the grocery store shelves is no longer "normal food"? Testing on rats has shown that when fed GMO food compared to non-GMO food, some rats developed smaller brains, livers, and testicles, while others developed enlarged pancreases and intestines, and they were at higher risk for infection and disease (Smith 2003). How do we know GMOs aren't causing similar health issues in humans? Can GMOs lead to disastrous consequences for our health and/or the environment? In *Seeds of Deception,* Jeffrey Smith poses this unique question.

Another theory for why GMOs are a health hazard is that these altered genetic structures trigger our immune systems. Our bodies can recognize regular tomatoes, but if those tomatoes are genetically modified and their structure has changed, our bodies may flag the alert to attack those foreign molecules. That may explain why food sensitivities and full-blown food allergies are on the rise along with autoimmune diseases. I can't tolerate any wheat in the United States, but I tried bread while on my honeymoon in Europe and I didn't have the same severe side effects that I do here. What was the difference? Europe doesn't allow GMOs (Bello 2013).

Chemicals in Soil

In chapter 4 I discussed why our soil is so deficient, due in part to herbicide and pesticide usage. Soil is another source of our toxin exposure. Some researchers even believe pesticides have entirely contaminated our air, water, and soil—and now us. Yikes! I've also previously mentioned the dangers of the herbicide atrazine. In Iowa, where I live, there is high exposure to this chemical, and there are high brain cancer rates (Williams 2014). Could there be an association?

Air Where You Live

Depending on the toxicity of the area in which you live, you may also be exposed to various toxins simply from air pollution. In my city, there are several factories daily polluting our air. The Scorecard website, www.scorecard.goodguide.com, lets you obtain more information on the pollution in your community with just a few clicks.

Electromagnetic Fields

How often have you assessed how much electromagnetic chaos and stress you are exposing your family to? Do you sleep with your cell phone inches from your head? Do you use Bluetooth devices? Does your baby—whose skull isn't fully developed—sleep a foot away from a wireless baby monitor? Wireless radiation can cause sterility. It can complicate cardiovascular conditions. It can lead to developmental delays. It depletes your body of antioxidants. It can impact your autonomic nervous systems (less EMF). Do you want to know more? *Full Signal* is an hour-long documentary on these dangers.

Tobacco and Alcohol

Lifestyle choices also contribute to toxic load. Do you smoke? If so, did you know that there are more than six hundred ingredients in cigarettes? When burned, these create more than seven thousand chemicals. At least sixty-nine are known to cause cancer, and many are poisonous (Lung.org 2017). Do you think your lungs rejuvenate in seven years and that your complications from smoking are now gone? Think again. I've seen high cadmium levels in patients who haven't smoked or been exposed to secondhand smoke for years. Cadmium also comes from battery acid. However, unless my patients worked in a battery factory, the likely source of exposure was cigarettes. Alcohol is another toxic lifestyle choice. When you drink alcohol, ammonia is created. Your liver helps convert ammonia to urea, which also has to be eliminated via the kidneys in urine. If your liver can't quite do the job, your levels of ammonia can rise.

Medications, Mercury, and Yes, Vaccines

Did you know ibuprofen contains heavy metals? Peel back the label and read the ingredients yourself. Over-the-counter (OTC) and prescription drugs and vaccinations are often full of toxic agents. They can contain heavy metals like aluminum and mercury. I don't want aluminum placed on my skin, let alone injected into my body. I certainly wouldn't want it injected into my child's body. Mercury is also a potent neurotoxin, but some people have a mouthful of it with their fillings—I've had mine removed. Vaccines can also contain aborted fetal tissue, formaldehyde (which is used as a preservative), antifreeze, ethanol, monosodium glutamate (MSG, an excitotoxin), latex—the list goes on and on (Hamborsky, Kroger, and Wolfe 2015). My hope is that vaccine manufacturers will eventually come to their senses and remove the suspicious ingredients. To learn more about vaccines, visit the National Vaccine Information Center, www.nvic.org. There have been several documentaries on this topic, one of which is *Vaxxed*, by Andrew Wakefield. I personally am pro informed choice, and think every individual should receive education on what chemicals they choose to put in their body, including those in vaccinations.

That Daily Jumpstart

What about your daily or weekly trip to the coffee shop? Coffee can also be toxic, so even this should be grown organically. To learn more about the common toxins found in coffee (like mold toxins), read *The Bulletproof Diet*, by Davis Asprey. I was shocked at how toxic coffee can be. Additionally, it is often drunk from a paper cup lined with plastic and capped with a plastic lid—two sources that can leach into the liquid and be consumed with every sip.

Personal Care Products

Are you a makeup junkie? For years, personal care products have been laced with chemicals that cause allergies, cancer, and endocrine disruptions. Parabens and phthalates are two well-known endocrine-disrupting chemicals (EDCs). EDCs have been implicated in neurological diseases, reproductive disorders, thyroid dysfunction, and immune and metabolic disorders. To learn more, visit the Endocrine Disruption Exchange.

The United States hasn't passed any legislation regarding the safety of the personal care industry since 1938, and that law was only one-and-a-half pages long. That means the fourteen hundred chemicals that Europe has banned are *still* being placed into our everyday shampoos, body lotions, and makeup. Did you know that often, the darker the makeup shades, the higher the heavy metal count? Lipsticks often contain lead. Perfumes and fragrances are really just words for nasty a blend of petrochemicals, which means "petrolatum-based," and bad news for you. Parabens are the most widely used preservatives in personal care products. They are used to stop fungus and bacteria from growing in your products. Phthalates are used to soften and increase the flexibility of plastic and vinyl. These chemicals can bind to our hormone receptors and cause disruption or interference with our hormone signaling.

Products in the Home

How do you clean your clothes and your home? Detergent, fabric softener, and oven cleaner all are extremely toxic. To learn more about the dangers of these chemicals, read *Toxin Free,* by Debra Lynn Dadd. Do you use air fresheners in your car? These contain phthalates, which, again, are cancer causing, and can also cause endocrine disruption.

Dry-Cleaned Clothes

Do you dry-clean your clothing? Wearing a newly cleaned suit can expose you to high levels of perchloroethylene (also known as trichloroethylene), which is likely carcinogenic (cancer causing) to humans (American Cancer Society 2014). When inhaled, this industrial solvent can cause central nervous system depression. It can also cause anesthesia, slowed heart rate, and unconsciousness. If you must dry-clean, at least take off the plastic and allow your clothes to air out in the garage before you bring them into your little closet to air out into your bedroom.

THE HUMAN BODY—ITS OWN SOURCE OF TOXICITY

How many states now have a population in which over 33 percent of its residents are obese? Too many. Toxins lead to obesity. Toxins hide in fat cells. Obesity leads to multiple chronic diseases. Could there be a link between toxicity and obesity? Detoxing certainly helps facilitate toxin release from fat cells, and then the fat cells can shrink. And detoxing promotes weight loss, which helps improve health. Interestingly, weight loss without proper detoxification causes toxins to be released from the fat cells into the blood stream where they can be continuously recirculated. So if you are pursuing weight loss consider trying a selective detox program, after, of course, making sure you have a strong and healthy foundation.

In addition to the role of fat cells in retaining toxins, the human body itself can be fairly toxic without optimal gut health. Carbohydrates ferment and proteins putrefy inside the body, making some pretty bad gas. If you are stressed and not working to heal your stressors—psychological or emotional—your body can remain in a toxic state.

Even the US Environmental Protection Agency (EPA) admits that 100 percent of the humans it has studied have chemical stores in their fat. These chemicals are potent cancer causers and include dioxins, polychlorinated biphenyls (PCBs), dichlorobenzene, and xylene.

According to the World Health Organization (WHO), dioxins are very toxic and cause reproductive and developmental problems. They can interfere with our hormones and cause cancer (WHO 2016).

PCBs are aromatic, synthetic, man-made chemicals that do not occur naturally in the environment. They are no longer commonly used due to their health hazards. Still, dioxins and PCBs outgas from copy paper, plastics, inks, paints, furnishings, flame retardants, foam, pads, and construction glues. Unfortunately, even though PCBs are not commonly used, they are still found in dairy and meat sources, because they have built up in our food chains thanks to bioaccumulation.

Bioaccumulation occurs when an organism absorbs a toxic substance faster than it can excrete it. Humans are at the top of the food chain, so if grains have been sprayed with pesticides, and animals consume the grains, and we eat the animals, we may not even know how many chemicals we have exposed ourselves to.

PLASTICS—THEY'RE EVERYWHERE

Yes, plastic is toxic and not meant to be ingested. Think of how often you use plastic on a daily basis—cough spray, baby formula, peanut butter, and ketchup, for example, all likely came in a plastic container. How do you know for sure that the plastic didn't leach from the container into your foods? Plastic often contains bisphenol A (BPA). This is an endocrine disruptor that can have negative effects on our reproductive organs and hormones, specifically the breasts in females and prostate in males. Currently, several states are in the process of adopting legislation to regulate the use of BPA in food and beverage containers and children's products.

Do you eat out of aluminum cans? You're not safe there, either. These also contain BPA, which may be leaching into your food. Glass is a safer choice than either plastic or aluminum.

Xylene is one of the top thirty chemical products in the United States. It is a solvent (a liquid that dissolves other substances) that outgasses from gasoline, printing, rubber, plastics, carpeting, furnishings, varnishes, construction materials, permanent markers, and industrial and traffic exhaust, even from airplane fuel.

Styrene outgasses from Styrofoam cups and takeout containers. It also outgasses from our computers and plastics. It is used extensively in the manufacturing of plastics, rubber, and resins. People who manufacture boats, tubs, and showers, are potentially exposed to styrene. Health effects from exposure to styrene may involve the central nervous system, and include complaints of headache, fatigue, dizziness, confusion, drowsiness, malaise, difficulty in concentrating, and a feeling of intoxication.

A toxic exposure study by the EPA titled the Wallace Study examined the exhaled breath of New Jersey residents and found numerous chemicals, including those listed above (Wallace 1987). Additionally, the average American has 116 of 148 synthetic compounds in their body at all times (Biomonitoring California 2005). These included the aforementioned dioxins, PCBs, and organochlorine pesticides. The study also revealed that these same substances were found in human milk, umbilical cord blood, the placenta, and the blood and body fat of newborn babies. In fact, the average umbilical cord blood contained 217 neurotoxins, 208 of which were known to cause birth defects. Everyone stores toxins, and they can be passed on to offspring.

Sick mommies make sick babies—so detox *before* you conceive. Do not detox if you are pregnant or nursing.

In 2015, the United Stated produced five hundred billion pounds of chemicals. What happens when the chemicals mix with water, air, food, or other chemicals? We have no idea what other toxins could arise. Of all the chemicals made, chemical combination has yet to be researched. Each year, the CDC announces a Toxic Release Inventory. "Certain industrial facilities in the US must report annually how much of each chemical is recycled, combusted for energy recovery, treated for destruction, and disposed of or otherwise released on- and off-site. This information is collectively referred to as production-related waste managed" (EPA 2015). According to the 2015 reported data, the United States had 27.2 billion pounds of chemical waste: 698.6 million pounds were emitted into the air, 191.1 million pounds into the water supply, and 2 billion pounds into the land. The data show that many toxic chemicals were released via air, water, and land across the United States. You can search by your zip code for a report in your area. Visit www.epa.gov/trinationalanalysis for a report for your area.

In Rachel Carson's book *Silent Spring*, she states, "For the first time in the history of the world, every human being is now subjected to contact with dangerous chemicals, from the moment of conception until death." Brenda Watson describes it in another way in her book *The Detox Strategy*, stating that we live in a "toxic soup" of dangerous chemicals. There's no escaping that truth.

SYMPTOMS OF TOXICITY

The US agencies—the National Institutes of Health and the CDC—admit that 60 to 80 percent of all diseases, including heart disease and cancer, is linked to environmental and lifestyle factors. How do you know if you are toxic? Try filling out the detox questionnaire at www.yourlongevityblueprint.com.

SIGNS THAT YOUR DETOXIFICATION CAPACITY MIGHT BE IMPAIRED

- ☐ Digestion, Elimination Problems *(constipation, bloating, diarrhea, nausea, heartburn)*
- ☐ Blood Sugar and Hormonal Imbalances
- ☐ Elevated Cholesterol
- ☐ PMS
- ☐ Overweight/Underweight
- ☐ Asthma
- ☐ Allergies
- ☐ Frequent Flus, Colds, Sinus Infections
- ☐ Skin Disorders
- ☐ Muscle and Joint Pain, Fibromyalgia
- ☐ Fatigue
- ☐ Insomnia
- ☐ Anger, Depression, Irritability
- ☐ Chemical Sensitivities

If you identify with many of the signs listed above, a portion of your impaired health may be due to inadequate clearance of toxins within the liver-gastrointestinal systems.

HOW OUR BODIES DETOXIFY

Now that I've discussed how toxic we likely all are, let me review the detoxification organs in the human body and how detoxing works.

Detoxification is a fancy word for how the body eliminates the waste it is exposed to and the waste created through normal bodily functions.

The **liver** is the primary organ for detoxification, because it filters the blood. It's a little like the washing machine for your body. It weighs roughly three pounds, and is one of the largest organs. It's found in the right upper abdomen under your ribs. The liver helps break down and clear steroid hormones, and it also breaks down fats to help produce energy. The liver produces a yellow/brown, sometimes green, liquid called **bile**, which is carried through the bile duct to the small intestines. It also helps to keep blood sugar levels constant despite the carbohydrates you eat. The liver removes sugar from the blood when needed and stores it in the form of glycogen. If blood sugar levels are low, the liver can release the sugar from glycogen. The liver also stores vitamins and minerals and releases them when needed. Blood is removed from the liver via three hepatic veins. The liver also assists in creating blood-clotting factors. The liver is smart. It helps to prevent the storage of fat-soluble toxins by turning them into water-soluble toxins that can be excreted.

The portal vein brings blood from the digestive system to the liver. This blood contains nutrients, toxins, and sometimes medications. In the liver, these substances are processed, stored, altered, detoxified, and passed back into the blood or released back into our bowels to be eliminated. The liver converts toxic substance into harmless waste to be excreted from the body. Your liver can, for example, remove alcohol from your blood and get rid of the end products of medications. The liver does this through two major phases. Phase 1 involves the cytochrome P450 enzymes, which, through several different processes, chemically changes fat-soluble toxins into intermediary metabolites. These are more toxic than the initial toxins. Many individuals experience headaches, nausea, and muscle aches when they undergo a detox program, because their phase 2 detox pathways aren't up to speed. Phase 2 involves conjugation or attachment of specific molecules onto the intermediary metabolites, rendering them nontoxic and water soluble so that they can be excreted through the urine, bile, or stool. In order for these pathways and processes to work, the liver requires nutrients such as the previously discussed B vitamins, glutathione, and amino acids. These nutrients are literally the fuel, the building blocks, for the liver to do what it is supposed to do. If toxins don't get excreted, they end up in storage.

Here are the nutrients your body needs to rid itself of chemicals.

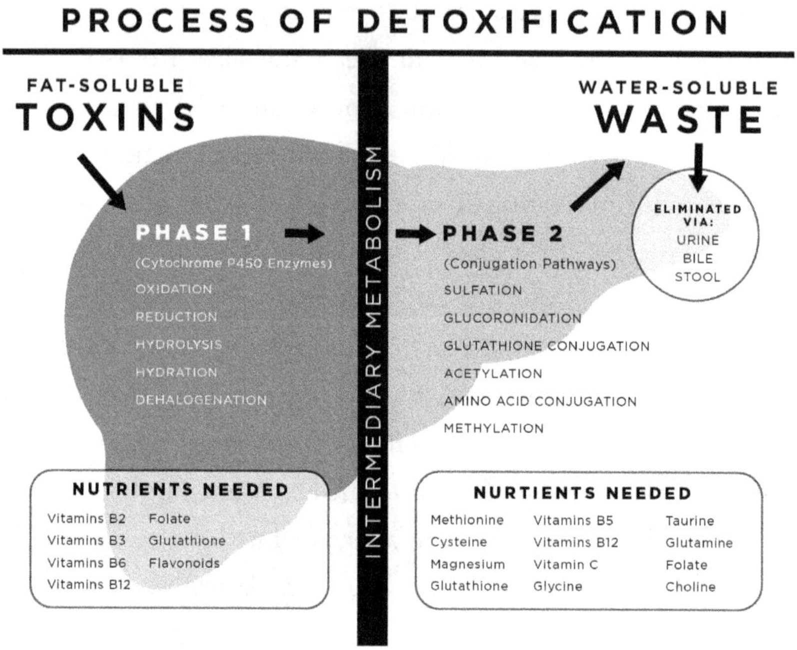

As Sherry Rogers, MD, says in her book *Detoxify or Die*, "The secret is in getting your body so chemically unloaded and nutrient primed, that it heals itself" (Rogers 2002). The best way to do this is to fix your nutritional deficiencies to get the detox pathways working well and then consider a liver detox program where your body will be provoked to dump its burden of toxins.

The drain pump that helps with that dump is your **gallbladder**. The gallbladder sits under the liver. It is mostly a storage organ that helps in the digestion of fats. It assists in making bile more concentrated. Bile travels from the liver to the gallbladder in channels called bile ducts. These ducts store the bile until it is released into the small intestine, where most absorption of fats takes place.

The **kidneys** play an important role in detoxing as well. Think of them as "waste collectors." Every day, your kidneys filter or process about two hundred quarts of blood to sift out about two quarts of waste products and extra water that become urine, which flows to your bladder through tubes called ureters. Your bladder then stores the urine until you go to the bathroom. This chapter primarily concerns our livers, but do not underestimate how important the kidneys are.

HOW TO REDUCE YOUR TOXIC LOAD

There are a number of ways to reduce your toxic load naturally:

HOW TO REDUCE YOUR TOXIN LOAD

1. QUIT POISONING YOURSELF
2. EAT ORGANIC
3. DRINK CLEAN WATER
4. PURIFY YOUR AIR
5. CLEAN UP YOUR HOME
6. INCORPORATE EARTHING/GROUNDING
7. CHOOSE GLASS OVER PLASTIC
8. CLEAN UP YOUR PERSONAL CARE PRODUCTS

DIRTY DOZEN

- APPLES
- CELERY
- STRAWBERRIES
- PEACHES
- SPINACH
- NECTARINES
- GRAPES
- SWEET BELL PEPPERS
- POTATOES
- BLUEBERRIES
- LETTUCE
- KALE

SOURCE: www.ewg.org

CLEAN 15

- SWEET CORN
- AVOCADOS
- PINEAPPLES
- CABBAGE
- ONIONS
- SWEET PEAS
- PAPAYAS
- ASPARAGUS
- MANGOS
- EGGPLANT
- HONEYDEW MELON
- KIWI
- CANTALOUPE
- CAULIFLOWER
- GRAPEFRUIT

SOURCE: www.ewg.org

Quit Poisoning Yourself

As Dr. Mark Hyman says, "Think about it, if there is a health food section in the grocery store, what does that make the rest of the food sold there?" Think about what you are putting into your body. Toxic foods do not nourish a healthy body. There is greater realization today that a high percentage of cancer is caused by diet and environment, two things you can change. Dr. Hyman also says, "I believe the most important and most powerful tool you have to change your health and the world is your fork." One major change you can make is to eat organic as often as you can. If you can't always purchase organic, at least buy organic versions of the "Dirty Dozen" foods, or wash the nonorganic versions well. The Dirty Dozen are thin-skinned foods that pesticides and herbicides can easily penetrate. The list includes apples, celery, strawberries, peaches, spinach, nectarines, grapes, sweet bell peppers, potatoes, blueberries, lettuce, and kale. Several companies, such as Norwex, offer a fruit and veggie cloth that can be used to help wipe off wax and other toxins caught within.

Drink Water—Lots of It

Drink half your body weight in ounces each day, but make sure you aren't drinking toxins. Clean up your water. Not just chemicals, but even pharmaceutical drugs have been found contaminating our water. Do you want to purchase fresh spring water? The Find a Spring website is a community and user-created database of natural springs around the world where you can pick up spring water. Make sure you use a filter for your shower as well as your drinking water. The Brita and Pur carbon filters are a great start. They will get rid of heavy metals, parasites, and pesticides. At my office, we have a machine that works beyond simple filtration. We use High Tech Health's water alkalinizer. It has a carbon filter to remove all bacteria. It filters out contaminants, metals, and chlorine. The water in the machine is also treated with electrolysis, which essentially ionizes the minerals, making them much more bioavailable, and much more hydrating. The alkaline water also contains more available stable oxygen and it becomes charged. This water has been written up in peer-reviewed journals as a superior antioxidant or free radical scavenger. Lastly, this water is treated with low-dose ultraviolet light to eliminate viruses (the bacteria has already been filtered out). The ultraviolet light remains on for thirty seconds after the water stops flowing to eliminate reverse contamination of the unit. The best feature about my machine? It will last twelve years (similar to many appliances). The price, including filter changes, works out to about fourteen cents per gallon— a small price to pay for the daily use of a water unit that will dramatically improve your family's health. If you are interested in purchasing a machine like this, visit High Tech Health's website, www.hightechhealth.com/products/water-electrolyzers, and use my name as a promo code for substantial savings.

Reverse Osmosis (RO) removes bad and good minerals. If you drink RO water, be sure to replete the minerals it has depleted you of. Also, don't drink out of plastic. Choose glass. We sell LifeFactory glass bottles at my clinic. Patients love them!

Clean Up Your Air

It's easy to underestimate the importance of air, but you can survive only three minutes without it. And, truth be told, you may be exposed to more toxins inside your house than out. The volatile organic compounds (VOCs) acetate, ethanol, and formaldehyde could be floating around your home. Do you use hairspray? Have you recently had your carpets cleaned? Even wood preservatives can outgas toxic chemicals. Consider adding live plants to your home to help filter the air. Invest in a high-quality air purifier like a high efficiency particle absorption (HEPA) filter. Clean the ducts in your house and change your filters often. You can also find top-rated air purifiers at AirPurifiers.com.

Clean Up Toxins in Your Home

Use a shower filter to filter out the chlorine. You spend one-third of your life in bed, so purchase an organic mattress and use organic cotton sheets. For many more ways to clean and clear toxins from where you live, read Debra Dadd's book *Toxic Free*, where she guides you through fifty steps to clean up your home. Her book is extremely thorough, with a quick-start guide for you to immediately start protecting your health by ridding your home of toxins. One tip she offers: leave your shoes at your door. Think of all the chemicals that lie on the soles of your shoes that you carry through your house and leave on your carpet, only to then walk barefoot over.

Get in Touch with Earth

In Clinton Ober, Stephen Sinatra, and Martin Zucker's book, *Earthing: The Most Important Health Discovery Ever?* the authors argue how humans are what they call very earth disconnected and earth starved. They teach you how important it is to ground yourself, to connect back to the earth. Walking on grass, the beach, the sidewalk, even on dirt helps you receive and become charged with electrons. This will help protect you against the dangerous oxidative free radicals from wireless radiation. Turn off your cell phone or put it in airplane mode as you sleep. Practice these grounding techniques and become more disconnected from electromagnetic chaos and more connected to the earth. Doing so, they explain, will help reduce inflammation, pain, and stress and improve blood flow, sleep, and energy.

Other Ways to Reduce Toxic Load

Choose glass over plastic for storage, drinking and cooking. **Avoid use of fluorescent bulbs**, which contain mercury. Think about every purchase you make. Is this a safe or toxic item? Do you want to bring it into your home?

Choose clean personal care products. It can be an overwhelming and difficult task to find safer products such as toothpaste without sodium lauryl sulfate or fluoride, or aluminum-free deodorant. But when it comes to cosmetics, two organizations are helping shed light on our products. The Environmental Working Group posts a safe cosmetics database that relies on voluntary participation from cosmetics makers. The organization also produces a Healthy Living App that allows you to scan your products to see how toxic they are. The Campaign for Safe Cosmetics, www.safecosmetics.com, is a coalition that educates the public on toxicity concerns and is working to pressure the cosmetics industry to make safer products. I personally use Beautycounter for cosmetics. Learn more at www.beautycounter.com/stephaniegray.

Use safe cleaning products as well. Many unique products can be found through Norwex. View their products at www.norwex.biz. As you transition to better products, please make sure you dispose of your household hazardous waste legally and safety. Find out where in your local community you can dispose of toxic chemicals.

HOW TO AID YOUR BODY IN DETOXIFICATION

Detoxify your body naturally by choosing to consume foods that promote detoxification. These include foods high in antioxidants; the more color the better. Pomegranates and blueberries are high in antioxidants, but spices are, too. Clove, cinnamon, oregano, turmeric, and basil actually have a higher value than those berries do. **ORAC** value stands for the Oxygen Radical Absorbance Capacity. It attempts to quantify the total antioxidant capacity (TAC). For foods highest in antioxidants, visit Superfoodly at www.superfoodly.com. Our high ORAC LB vegetable antioxidant blend is called Super Greens.

Incorporate into your diet sulfur-based foods like greens, kale, chard, and cabbage as well as mushrooms (unless you need to avoid fungus/yeast). Add in algae, spirulina, or chlorella to your smoothie or salad, as these can help bind heavy metals. Add garlic, which boosts glutathione, and cilantro, which helps bind heavy metals, to as many meals as you can. Parsley is a weak diuretic that helps the kidneys. Consider superfoods like Moringa powder, which helps with detoxification. Beets and artichokes stimulate bile flow.

Keep your bowels regular. You should be having one or more unforced bowel movements every day. If you are not, examine your water intake. You must drink lots of water to keep your body hydrated. Hydration is also essential to detoxification and for supporting your kidneys to remove the water-soluble toxins.

Have you heard of colonics? Colon hydrotherapy (also known as high enemas or colon irrigation) is a procedure where purified water is washed into the large intestine to clean and remove built-up fecal matter. This can be incredibly helpful for patients with chronic constipation. I've also seen it help patients lose weight as it helped them excrete built-up waste. To learn more, visit the International Association for Colon Hydrotherapy at www.i-act.org.

Oil pulling has also become a popular way to detox. Oil pulling is the practice of swishing oils, often coconut oil, in the mouth to pull out impurities.

Get your lymphatics moving. Your lymphatics carry toxins out of your cells. Exercising helps with lymphatic drainage. Other activities to help include jumping on a small trampoline (known as rebounding), riding horses, and dry brushing. Dry brushing is great to perform before hopping into the shower. Dry brushing helps to unclog pores and get rid of toxins. Step-by-step instructions can be easily found on the internet.

Also, consider lymphatic drainage with a certified specialist. I know what it's like to struggle with toxicity. I had a lump in my left axilla, probably due to aluminum in my deodorant. I had several ultrasounds and was told everything was "normal." Disagreeing, I went to a lymphatic drainage specialist, who was able to get rid of the problem. She was able to immediately find this area and drain it. It was amazing. Conventional medicine had no other option for me than to wait until the lump was big enough to surgically remove. No, thank you. Lymph drainage was very helpful, comfortable, affordable, and successful for me.

Consider purchasing an infrared sauna. There are so many different sauna companies out there, and it can be difficult to determine which has the best quality. I personally use High Tech Health's dry far infrared sauna. Sunlighten is another brand I support. High Tech Health's sauna has proven detoxification results. Far infrared is a band of light (not visible) that is created by the sun and is felt as warmth on the body. Far infrared is effective because it penetrates deep into the body to elevate the body's core temperature, inducing a low-grade, short-term fever that helps with numerous health conditions. As far infrared is absorbed by the body's tissues, resonant absorption occurs. When the frequency of the far infrared matches the frequency of the water in your cells, that's when the magic happens. This activity causes toxins to be mobilized, releasing them from fat cells and dropping them into the blood, where they will be excreted via stool, urine, or sweat. High Tech Health has actually conducted trials looking at sweat samples showing all the harmful heavy metals that were released during the sauna session. These include aluminum, arsenic, cadmium, lead, and mercury. Sweating has also been shown to help remove phthalates and plastics, PCBs, dioxins, and pesticides. Saunas are also excellent for my patients who can't exercise due to mobility issues. It is a way for them to still get their heart rate up and sweat. To learn more about infrared sauna therapy, visit the High Tech Health's website, www.hightechhealth.com, and use my name for substantial savings. Also consider reading *No Sweat, Know Sweat,* by Bill Akpinar.

How many metal fillings are in your mouth? It is now illegal to put metal fillings in children's teeth. If you have metal fillings, with every chew you could be exposed to mercury vapors. See an environmental dentist who can help assess and safely remove metal from your mouth.

Find an acupuncturist who can help assess your liver and gallbladder function and promote the functioning of those organs. Also consider a personalized liver cleanse program. We offer Longevity Blueprint Core Restore one- and two-week beginners detox programs. Check out our video on this detoxification program at www.yourlongevityblueprint.com.

TESTING FOR TOXINS

Testing is not required prior to detoxing. I often detox patients without testing. However, there are times that we need to know what toxins are elevated in patients to help us personalize their treatments. For every person, the rate and places of storage can vary. For some individuals, toxins hide in bone, others in the liver, some in muscles, milk, or semen, and others even in the brain.

The nutritional analysis shows basic levels of heavy metals. If any heavy metals flag as high, I often then pursue more specific testing with my patients. Several labs exist that offer testing for heavy metals. I most commonly use a urine toxic metals test through Doctors Data. To help assess toxicity, retention is assessed. Patients are given a chelation or binding agent to mobilize stored metals from fat. Levels are checked before and after the patient is given a chelation agent. If levels return high after taking the agent, it is assumed that the patient has high levels of toxins in their body.

Some patients have brought me hair analysis in the past to review for them. Some toxic elements are more concentrated in the hair than blood or urine, and there is a time and place for hair testing. However, a lot of my patients dye their hair, which then skews the test results. This is one of the main reasons I typically don't rely on hair testing alone.

If I specifically want to assess mercury, Quicksilver Scientific offers a Mercury Tri-Test, which is a combination of blood, hair, and urine testing. They describe their test as utilizing mercury speciation analysis, a "patented advanced technology that **separates methyl mercury (MeHg) from inorganic mercury (HgII) and measures each directly**." What this means is that they can differentiate where the mercury source is coming from, fish versus metal fillings in your mouth.

When looking for toxic chemicals, I typically use the Great Plains Laboratory. They have a test, the GPL-TOX, which is a toxic nonmetal chemical profile that screens for the presence of 172 different toxic chemicals, some of which I've mentioned, including "organophosphate pesticides, phthalates, benzene, xylene, vinyl chloride, pyrethroid insecticides, acrylamide, perchlorate, diphenyl phosphate, ethylene oxide, acrylonitrile, and more."

The Great Plains Laboratory also has a test looking for toxic levels of glyphosate. Glyphosate is the world's most widely produced herbicide and is the primary toxic chemical in Roundup and many other herbicides. These tests should only be conducted under the supervision of an experienced provider who can help you interpret the results.

SUPPLEMENTS TO HELP WITH DETOXING

The exact same detox program won't be used on everyone. Again, it's important to note that detoxing is *not* for women who are pregnant or nursing. Ideally, detox before conceiving. If you have diabetes, please consult with your health care provider. Also, do not detox if you have acute appendicitis or gallbladder or liver disease. If your condition is chronic, do not detox without supervision from an experienced provider.

The nutrients listed on the previous graph are necessary for the liver to work effectively. Think of these nutrients as the soap. When you do laundry, your clothes can't get clean without soap. In your body, you must have adequate glutathione for your detox pathways to work well. I often supplement my patients with this nutrient, a need I can test for with a nutritional evaluation.

A comprehensive detoxification program will provide nutrients to the patient with a protein powder often containing fiber and bentonite clay to help bind toxins the body has. I have my patients also abide by a modified fast the first few days of the liver detox. As the week progresses, we add the lipotropics, choleretics, and cholagogues.

Lipotropics help break fat down and transport it out of the liver. These include methionine, choline, and inositol, as well as choleretics and cholagogues, which are herbs that help increase production and excretion of bile. These include beets, artichoke, yellow dock, and dandelion. Nearly every liver detox program that I have used also uses silymarin (milk thistle). It has several liver protection benefits, is an antioxidant and antiviral, and has anti-inflammatory properties.

Our Core Restore liver detox program uses a protein/fiber/bentonite clay powder to bind toxins and help you eliminate them, as well as a comprehensive multivitamin with nutrients needed for detoxification, and a product called Liver Detox, which contains the lipotropics, choleretics, and cholagogues. You can view instructions for our basic seven-day Core Restore program at www.yourlongevityblueprint.com.

If it is found that a patient has severe heavy metal toxicity, appropriate chelation agents can be used to help chelate or to bind the heavy metal so that it can be excreted from the body. For instance, calcium EDTA may be used to bind or chelate cadmium, DMPS/DMSA may be used to bind mercury, and a combination of EDTA and DMSA may be used to bind lead. Chelation can be given orally, rectally, or intravenously. Chelation should only be done through a provider who is certified and very experienced. This is only for patients with normal kidney function.

CONCLUSION

Scott, the car mechanic from the beginning of this chapter, took my words very seriously. He realized his body wasn't able to rid itself of the toxins he continued to expose himself to on a daily basis. Not only did he change jobs to reduce his exposure (which I realize to some may seem extreme), but he followed a two-month liver detox program and then completed an additional liver/gallbladder flush several times. He followed my advice word for word and had incredible results. When he returned for his follow-up visit, the list of foods he could consume without reacting had greatly increased, and his list of sensitivities had declined. His SIBO didn't return. His emotional state had improved. His anxiety was entirely gone. His energy and mental clarity were the highest he could remember in years. He had made a commitment to his health, preserving it and revitalizing it.

Just like how it's important to change your air filters or oil in your car several times each year, you should be working to revitalize your liver and, in essence, change its filter. I recommend my patients undergo our Core Restore liver detox program at least twice a year. You can detox your body following your Longevity Blueprint program.

When our bodies stop functioning the way we want them to, we often turn to the fireman approach—to conventional medicine, in other words. Instead, we should be looking to remove the toxic chemicals from our bodies, homes, and environments. Every minute of life, your laundry room—your liver, gallbladder, and kidneys—is working hard to purify and detoxify your body. As with your laundry in the home, detoxing is ongoing for the body. You can work to reduce your toxic exposure, and you can work to revitalize your detoxification organs like your liver, so that your body can handle the incoming burden of toxins. You get to choose to take advantage of this powerful information. You get to choose to live a toxic-free life.

Longevity Blueprint Nutraceutical Products

Here are my favorite LB nutrients:

- Core Restore Liver Detox Kit
- Liver Cleanse Support
- Liver Detox
- Super Greens

- Antioxidant Support
- NAC

Chapter 5 Resources

AirPurifiers.com: www.airpurifiers.com/

Beautycounter: www.beautycounter.com/stephaniegray

Bulletproof Coffee information: http://www.bulletproof.com/

Campaign for Safe Cosmetics: www.safecosmetics.org

The Endocrine Disruption Exchange: https://.endocrinedisruption.org

Environmental Working Group: www.ewg.org

Environmental Working Group Healthy Living App (to scan personal care products for toxicity): www.ewg.org/apps

Find A Spring: www.findaspring.com

Full Signal documentary: http://fullsignalmovie.com

High Tech Health International: www.hightechhealth.com (use code **Stephanie Gray** to receive substantial savings)

International Association for Colon Hydrotherapy: www.i-act.org

The EMF Safety SuperStore: www.lessemf.org

Glass water bottles: https://www.lifefactory.com/

Living Downstream documentary: www.livingdownstream.com

Living Toxic Free website: www.debralynndadd.com

Norwex safe home cleaning products: http://norwex.biz/en_US/

National Vaccine Information Center: www.nvic.org

Score (pollution information site): http://scorecard.goodguide.com/

Sunlighten Sauna Company: www.sunlighten.com

Superfoodly: www.superfoodly.com

Vaxxed documentary: http://vaxxedthemovie.com/

International Academy of Oral Medicine and Toxicology: https://iaomt.org/

Top Air Purifiers: www.airpurifiers.com

Laboratories

Doctor's Data: www.doctorsdata.com

Quicksilver Scientific: www.quicksilverscientific.com/testing/mercury-tri-test

The Great Plains Laboratory: www.greatplainslaboratory.com/gpl-tox

Chapter 5 References

1. American Lung Association. "What's in a Cigarette?" Lung.org, (2017). http://www.lung.org/stop-smoking/smoking-facts/whats-in-a-cigarette.html?referrer=https://www.google.com.
2. Baker, Sidney MacDonald. *Detoxification and Healing: The Key to Optimal Health*. New Canaan, Connecticut: Keats Publishing Inc, 1997.
3. Bello, John and Foreign Policy in Focus. "Twenty-Six Countries Ban GMOs—Why Won't the US?" *The Nation* (October 2013). https://www.thenation.com/article/twenty-six-countries-ban-gmos-why-wont-us/.
4. Biomonitoring California. "Third National Report on Human Exposure to Environmental Chemicals." biomonitoring.ca.gov (2005). https://biomonitoring.ca.gov/downloads/third-national-report-human-exposure-environmental-chemicals-july-2005.
5. Carson, Rachel. *Silent Spring*. New York: First Mariner Books, 2002.
6. Dadd, Debra Lynn. *Toxic Free*. New York: Penguin Books, 2011.
7. "Dioxins and their effects on human health" World Health Organization (2016). Accessed August 25, 2017, http://www.who.int/mediacentre/factsheets/fs225/en.

8. LessEMF. "EMF and Infertility." LessEMF.com. https://www.lessemf.com/fertility.html.

9. Hamborsky, Jennifer, Andrew Kroger, and Charles Wolfe. *Epidemiology and Prevention of Vaccine-Preventable Diseases*. The Communication and Education Branch, National Center for Immunization and Respiratory Diseases, Centers for Disease Control and Prevention, (April 2015). https://www.cdc.gov/vaccines/pubs/pinkbook/downloads/table-of-contents.pdf.

10. Ober, Clinton, Stephen Sinatra, and Martin Zucker. *Earthing: The Most Important Health Discovery Ever?* Laguna Beach, California: Basic Health Publications, 2014.

11. Rogers, Sherry. *Detoxify or Die*. Sarasota, Florida: Sand Key Company, 2002.

12. Smith, Jeffrey. *Seeds of Deception*. Yes! Books, (2003).

13. Somers, Suzanne. *Sexy Forever: How to Fight Fat After Forty*. New York: Three Rivers Press, 2010.

14. US Environmental Protection Agency. "Toxic Release Inventory (TRI) National Analysis." EPA.gov (2015). https://www.epa.gov/trinationalanalysis.

15. Wallace, Lance. "The toxic exposure assessment methodology (team) study: Summary and analysis," vol. 1, U.S. Environmental Protection Agency (1987): 6–87. Accessed on the National Service Center for Environmental Publications (NSCEP) website, https://nepis.epa.gov.

16. Watson, Brenda. *The Detox Strategy*. New York: First Press, 2008.

17. Williams, Sean. "10 States Where Cancer Incidence Is The Highest." The Motley Fool (February 2014). https://www.thenation.com/article/twenty-six-countries-ban-gmos-why-wont-us/.

18. World Health Organization. "Dioxins and their effects on human health." WHO.int (2016). http://www.who.int/mediacentre/factsheets/fs225/en.

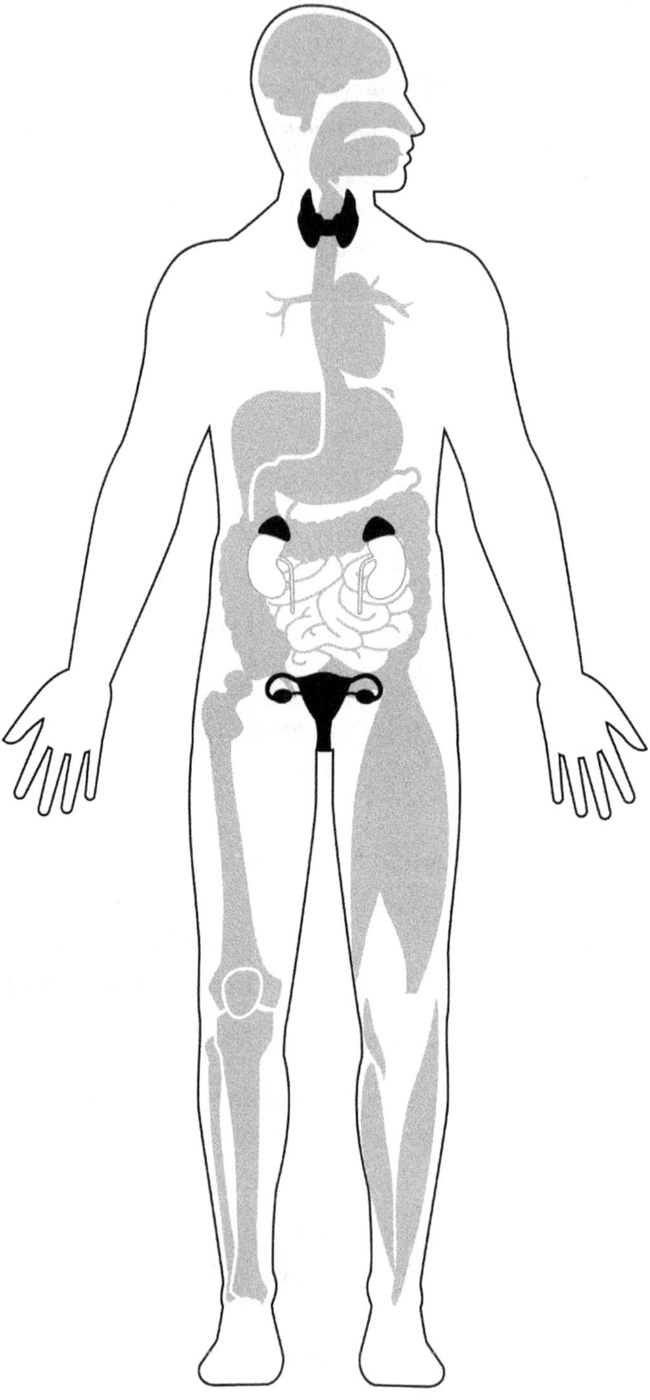

CHAPTER 6

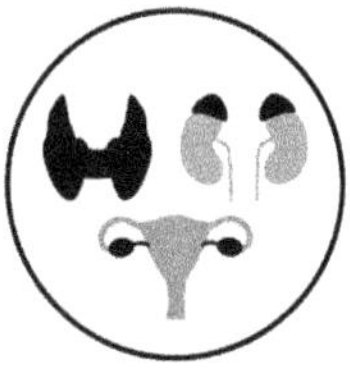

MANAGING YOUR HEATING/ COOLING: OPTIMIZING YOUR HORMONES

"Untreated hormone imbalances can have serious consequences, including osteoporosis, obesity, and breast cancer. Clearly, it's important to tune the body's hormones to their optimal levels, both individually and in relation to each other."

—Sara Gottfried, MD

In your home, during the hot and cold months, your comfort likely depends on the ability of your heating and cooling systems to regulate the temperature of the house.

Similarly, your body's comfort depends on its ability to heat and cool as needed. That's the role of your **endocrine system**, a network of glands that secrete hormones that are chemical messengers coordinating a range of bodily functions. If your thyroid isn't functioning properly, your fingertips may be cold, your metabolism may be sluggish, and you may feel like your internal furnace isn't kicking in. Conversely, if your sex hormone levels are low, you may feel like you are burning up inside, experiencing daily hot flashes and night sweats.

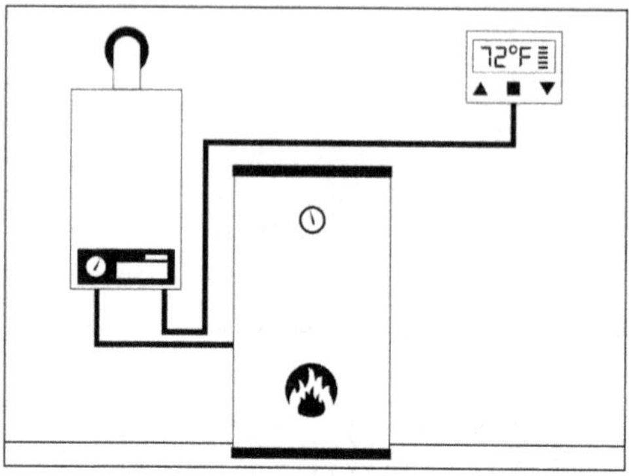

Think of your endocrine system as the heating and cooling system in your body. When your heating and cooling system isn't working—when your hormones are not balanced—you don't feel well. Every week, patients tell me how conventional medicine has failed them, how my functional medicine practice is their last resort, and how they desperately want to find a provider who will actually assess and treat their suspected hormone condition. Every week, a patient tells me: "I know I have a hormone issue, but my doctor checked all my hormones and he told me I'm normal. He wanted to give me an antidepressant. I know I'm not depressed. Please help me."

Gina was no different. She had a hysterectomy at twenty-eight years of age for heavy bleeding and endometriosis. Sadly, no provider offered to check her hormones or give her hormone replacement therapy until it was discovered that she had osteoporosis in her forties. Only then did one provider offer her synthetic hormone replacement therapy. At age forty-five, she finally visited my clinic. Up to that point, she had been taking oral Premarin, which helped her hot flashes but didn't help her sleep, energy, or libido. She was emotional and felt like she had been falling apart since her thirties. Additionally, she had been on synthetic thyroid replacement therapy without ever having had comprehensive thyroid levels tested. She had been told her thyroid levels were normal. But, after testing, she and I both disagreed, and together we got her on a better path, our Longevity Blueprint.

Cynthia had terrible depression and anxiety, and had experienced what some may call a nervous meltdown or breakdown. She had been given the runaround by several providers who didn't seem to know what to do with her. She had been suicidal and trialed on handfuls of antipsychotic medications until she found our clinic. All that time, medication was not helping her. Instead, it was making her worse, setting her up for unnecessary side effects and even withdrawal if she didn't take them exactly as prescribed. She often felt drugged up, and was unable to enjoy her life and her grandchildren. Sadly, assessing her, we found that her endocrine system had been neglected by conventional medicine and her hormone levels were terribly low as well.

HORMONES AND THE ENDOCRINE SYSTEM

I love helping patients optimize their hormones. In this chapter, I'll first discuss the three most important sex hormones: estrogen, progesterone, and testosterone. Then I'll discuss the adrenal and thyroid hormones and examine their relationship.

As I mentioned earlier, the endocrine system is a network of glands that secrete hormones, which are chemical signals coordinating a range of bodily functions. Think of a hormone as a chemical messenger made by a gland that acts to control certain actions of cells and organs. Essentially, hormones work in a key-and-lock fashion.

The endocrine system helps to regulate and control the following internal processes and systems:

- growth and development
- homeostasis (the internal balance of body systems)
- metabolism (body energy levels)
- reproduction
- response to stimuli (stress and/or injury)

The **hypothalamus** and **pituitary** work together in the brain. Think of your pituitary as the "furnace" in your home. It's controlled by the hypothalamus, or the "thermostat." The hypothalamus is about the size of an almond, and is located below the thalamus (a part of the brain that relays sensory information) and above the pituitary gland and brain stem.

The hypothalamus is the portion of the brain that maintains the body's internal balance, which is called homeostasis. It regulates things like your heart rate, blood pressure, electrolyte balance, appetite, and weight. The hypothalamus is the link between the endocrine and nervous systems. Many hormones are secreted by the hypothalamus. It also controls hormone production by releasing different chemicals to the pituitary.

The pituitary is a smaller, pea-sized gland located at the base of the brain. Remember that the hypothalamus signals the pituitary gland to stimulate or inhibit hormone production. These two are connected by the pituitary stalk, called the infundibulum. The pituitary hormones control other parts of the endocrine system, such as the adrenal and thyroid glands, ovaries, and testes.

The anterior pituitary gland secretes several hormones including prolactin, growth hormone, and adrenocorticotropic hormone (ACTH), which stimulates the adrenal glands to produce hormones. It also secretes follicle-stimulating hormones (FSH), and lutenizing hormones (LH). These help the ovaries and testes function normally. The pituitary also produces thyroid-stimulating hormones (TSH), which stimulates the thyroid gland to produce hormones.

Over the years, I've had several patients with pituitary tumors. If an individual has very low hormone levels, then it's possible that the pituitary is not working appropriately. The easiest way to check this is by ordering a prolactin level in the blood. High prolactin levels suggest a pituitary issue. If a prolactin level is high, I may order a brain scan for a pituitary tumor or refer the patient to an endocrinologist to determine if there is a hypothalamic or pituitary disorder.

FEMALE HORMONE PRODUCTION AND MENOPAUSE

Men and women both can have hormone imbalances, but the most commonly discussed hormone-related change for a woman is **menopause,** and for men is **andropause** (not "man-o-pause"). Why do menopause and andropause matter? People are now living longer; a hundred years ago, menopause was the end of a woman's lifespan; fifty years ago, women lived twenty years after menopause. Now, the postmenopause and postandropause life has increased by thirty-plus years, which is 40 to 50 percent of lifespan. We want to optimize those thirty-plus years (Donovitz 2015).

Many women think they will only experience hot flashes and night sweats for a few months. That isn't always the case. Usually by the time they have lost sleep for over a year they're ready to seek help balancing their hormones. However, I have seen female patients in their eighties and nineties who are still experiencing menopause symptoms that no one has been able to help.

If you haven't experienced menopause or andropause, you are in luck—there may still be time to improve your hormone function before you get there. Menopause doesn't just happen overnight. The Mayo Clinic states, "Menopause is the time that marks the end of your menstrual cycles. It's diagnosed after you've gone twelve months without a menstrual period. Menopause can happen in your forties or fifties, but the average age is fifty-one in the United States" (Mayo 2017). Menopause happens as the ovarian hormones decline. Eggs become depleted, thus ending the ability to reproduce.

Unfortunately, women often are symptomatic long before they are finished menstruating. This transitional period, called **perimenopause**, can take three to seven years. In perimenopause, the ovaries begin to decline, leading to lower hormone levels. That is why women start to have irregular cycles and become symptomatic. In these months to years, symptoms can include menstrual irregularity, increased PMS symptoms, bloating, water retention, vaginal dryness, low libido, acne, migraines, depression, mood changes, fatigue, thinning hair, sleep disturbances, hot flashes, night sweats, weight gain, and infertility.

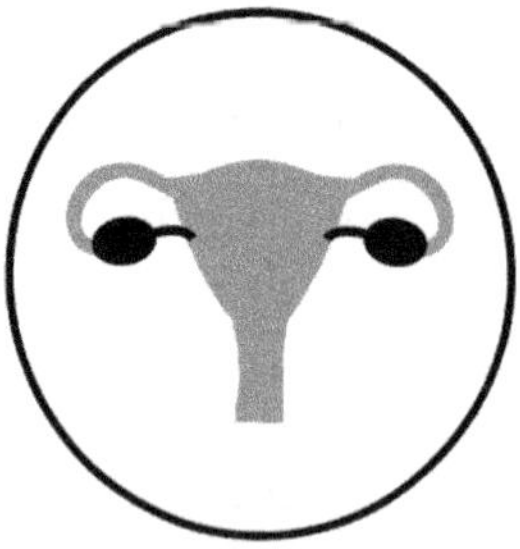

FEMALE HORMONE PRODUCTION AND MENOPAUSE

Sex hormones are primarily made in premenopausal women by the **ovaries**. The ovaries are small glandular organs about the shape and size of an almond. They are located on opposite sides of the uterus in the pelvic cavity and are attached to the uterus by the ovarian ligament. The ovaries are the most important organs of the female reproductive system. As glands, they secrete two major hormones, estrogen and progesterone.

Estrogen

Estrogen is one of the primary female sex hormones. It helps women maintain a youthful, feminine appearance, maintains memory and cognition, balances body temperature, and regulates sleep cycles. Estrogen assures healthy development of female sex characteristics such as breast development and fat distribution on the legs and hips during puberty. Estrogen also ensures fertility. As gonads, the ovaries produce eggs in women.

A lack of estrogen can cause hot flashes, night sweats, insomnia, poor concentration, smaller breasts, wrinkling skin, and dull hair and nails. During puberty, estrogen controls the development of the mammary glands and the uterus, and also helps stimulate the development of the uterine lining during the menstrual cycle. You may be surprised to find out you have three estrogens: **estrone**, **estradiol**, and **estriol**, all of which should be assessed.

You may have heard the term "estrogen dominance." Many providers do not believe in this, yet once they start examining hormone levels in patients, they quickly change their minds. Because of endocrine disruptors in our environment, we are now seeing many women with high estrogen and lower **progesterone**. This imbalance sets these women up for weight gain, fibroids, cysts, irregular bleeding, and potential risk of cancer.

Progesterone

Progesterone is another main female sex hormone, and it works to balance the effects of estrogen. Estrogen is a proliferative hormone, meaning it causes growth of tissue such as the uterine lining. Progesterone is anti-proliferative or antigrowth. This is another reason you do not want to be estrogen dominant. When the estrogen-to-progesterone ratio gets out of control, women may face an increased risk of breast or uterine cancer, fibroids, or endometriosis. Progesterone also helps to regulate the menstrual cycle, and having low levels of progesterone can lead to increased PMS, amenorrhea, infertility, and dysmenorrhea. Regarding reproduction, once the egg is released, progesterone levels rise. Progesterone acts on the uterus during pregnancy to allow the embryo to implant and develop in the womb.

Progesterone levels start to decline in women generally starting in their thirties. This is why so many young women experience PMS symptoms as well as anxiety and mood disturbances.

Progesterone is the first hormone I typically need to prescribe and optimize in younger women. I have found that the large majority of my perimenopausal patients who are taking sleep and/or anxiety medications have low progesterone. I've seen several extreme cases where women are heavily medicated yet are still having symptoms because no one has ever found and fixed their low progesterone problem. In many of these cases, once progesterone levels are improved, these individuals are weaned off their sleeping and anxiety medications. High progesterone is extremely rare. The main symptom I see in my patients with progesterone issues is moodiness.

In a normal twenty-eight-day menstrual cycle, the first two weeks are called the follicular phase. Here estrogen peaks with ovulation, then drops. Progesterone is then dominant during the last two weeks of the cycle.

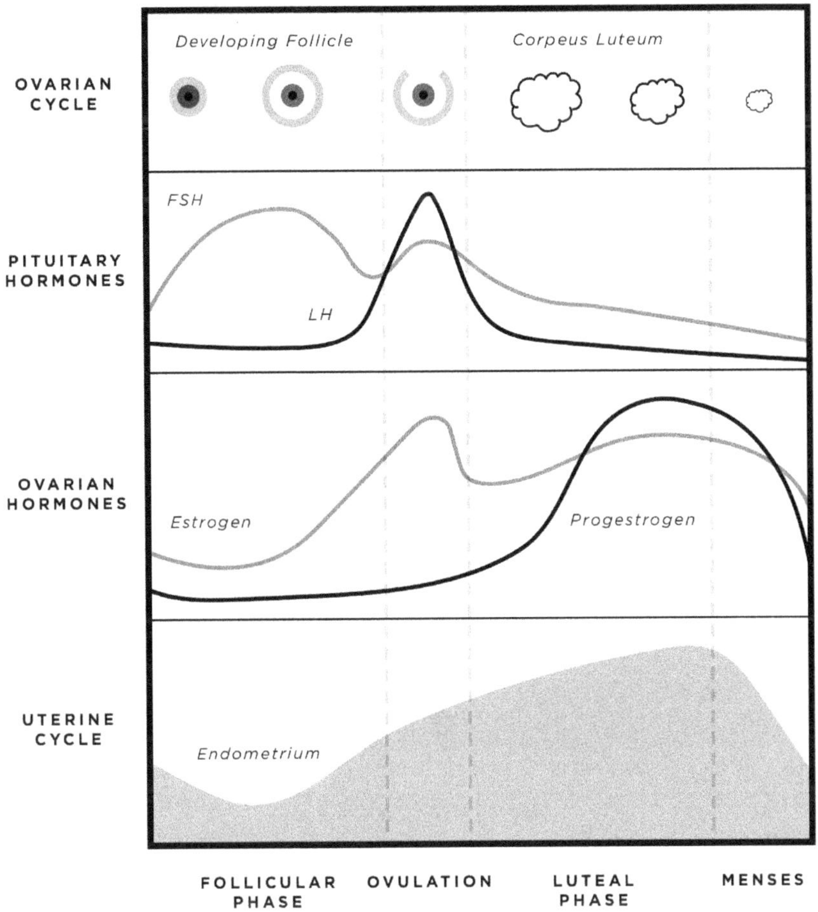

Testosterone

Testosterone helps with mood, motivation, drive, libido, energy, and muscle mass. Low testosterone can lead to fatigue, depression, muscle loss, poor exercise performance and stamina, reduced libido, thinning hair, and bone density challenges.

High testosterone can be found in women with **polycystic ovarian syndrome (PCOS)**. This is one of the most common hormone disorders in women. Symptoms include irregular or absent cycles, weight gain, fatigue, unwanted hair growth on the face, chest, and abdomen, known as hirsutism, thinning hair on the head, acne, pelvic pain, sleep and mood changes, headaches, and infertility. Early diagnosis can help reduce future risk, as PCOS has been linked to insulin resistance, type 2 diabetes, high cholesterol, high blood pressure, and heart disease. Combining symptoms with labs is the most comprehensive way to diagnose these patients.

REPRODUCTIVE SYSTEM

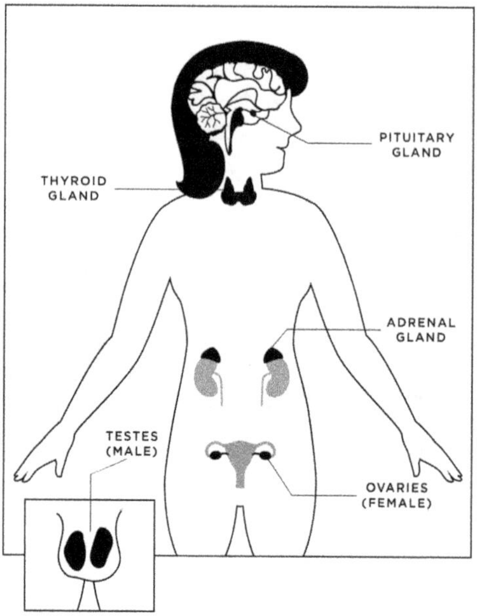

MALE HORMONE PRODUCTION AND ANDROPAUSE

The **testes** are the primary reproductive endocrine organs in men. They are twin, oval-shaped organs around the size of a large grape. They are located within the scrotum, a loose pouch of skin that hangs outside the body behind the penis. They work as glands to secrete testosterone, which is necessary for physical development of male characteristics. As gonads, they produce gametes or sperm in men.

During puberty, testosterone helps to transition a boy to manhood through development of male sex organs, increase in height and muscle mass, growth of facial and body hair, lowering of the voice, and growth of the Adam's apple. In adulthood, testosterone maintains libido, sperm production, muscle strength, and bone density.

Testosterone is produced through a network of feedback mechanisms. The hypothalamus sends a signal to the pituitary gland (both in the brain) to release a gonadotrophic follicle stimulating hormone (FSH), and a luteinizing hormone (LH). Luteinizing hormones stimulate testosterone production. If too much testosterone is produced, the hypothalamus alerts the pituitary gland to make less LH, which tells the testes to decrease testosterone levels and vice versa.

Andropause, or male menopause, is more common than you think. With andropause, the testicular production of testosterone starts to decline. This decline can generally begin in men in their thirties. Men typically lose 1 percent of their testosterone production each year. If they start declining in their thirties, they may feel lousy by the time they hit fifty. Hypogonadism is the name for clinically low testosterone.

The most common symptoms I see men seeking help for are low libido and erectile dysfunction (ED). By the time a man is experiencing ED, he likely has very low testosterone and has had it for a very long time. Other symptoms of low testosterone include fatigue, depression, muscle atrophy, weakness, poor exercise performance, reduced endurance, hair loss, weight gain, anxiety, and apathy. When I examine my patients, I also look for lack of hair growth on the legs, as this absence is a sign of low testosterone. Other physical symptoms of low testosterone are loss of body scent (pheromones), gynecomastia (man boobs), increased abdominal fat, poor muscle tone, male pattern baldness, and an underdeveloped beard (Hertoghe 2010).

Women aren't the only ones susceptible to bone loss, which I discussed in chapter 2. I've also seen men with osteoporosis and low testosterone who needed and benefited from hormone replacement.

In my practice, we encourage new male patients to fill out the male hormone questionnaire. This also helps provide them insight into how their symptoms could be related to low testosterone. The questionnaires can also be used to help patients track their improvement.

Female and male symptoms checklists are located on my clinic website, at www.ihhclinic.com.

ENDOCRINE DISRUPTORS

While patients are very thankful to finally have their hormones optimized, many ask why we now need hormone replacement therapy when generations ago we did not. I believe that is in part due to the toxic world we now live in that previous generations did not.

The escalating rate of cancer in the United States is in part due to constant exposure to toxic chemicals. Exposure to chemicals in the environment can increase the risk for hormone imbalances and hormone-related cancers. In large part, this is due to the endocrine-disrupting properties of these chemicals, which can trigger hormone responses that cause imbalances.

In the last chapter, I discussed endocrine-disrupting chemicals (EDCs), those compounds and chemicals found in the environment and in our products that we use on a daily basis and that have a direct impact on our endocrine systems. These non-natural, foreign-structured chemicals can block hormones, mimic their actions, and interfere with their function. Some of the most toxic endocrine disruptors include bisphenol A (BPA) from plastics, dioxins, phthalates, lead, and fire retardants, the latter of which can disrupt thyroid hormones. Even pesticides, herbicides, pollution, and personal care products can contain these EDCs.

Another reason many of my patients are dependent on hormone replacement therapy is because they underwent certain types of surgery. For instance, many of my patients have had partial or complete hysterectomies, which is the removal of a woman's ovaries, uterus and cervix. Many of these women were young—in their twenties and thirties. These women likely have had endocrine disruption and terrible hormone symptoms prior to their surgeries. Unfortunately, since they have come to me post-surgery, they no longer have the organs necessary to produce hormones. For optimal quality of life, they're now dependent on taking them as replacement therapy.

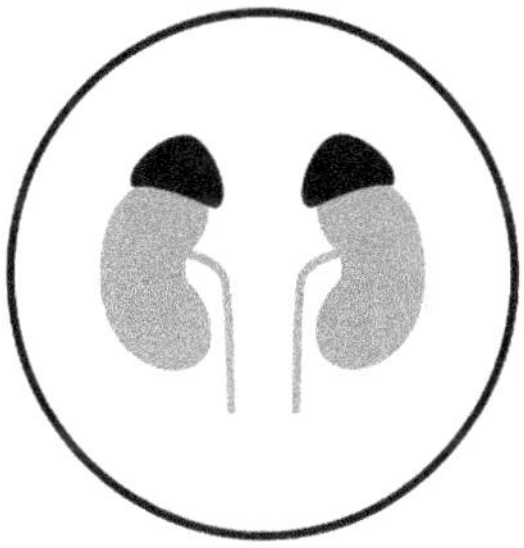

ADRENAL GLANDS, CORTISOL, AND NEUROTRANSMITTER PRODUCTION

The **adrenal glands** are two triangular glands one-and-a-half by three inches in size, located on top of your kidneys. Each of the glands is composed of two parts. The outer adrenal cortex produces essential hormones like cortisol (which helps regulate metabolism and helps your body respond to stress) and aldosterone (which helps maintain balance of salt and control blood pressure). The inner adrenal medulla produces hormones, including adrenaline. The release of these hormones is triggered by the hypothalamus and pituitary glands. The adrenals also help to a small degree with production of sex hormones, although the ovaries and testes are the primary producers (EndocrineWeb 2017). However, after menopause and andropause, the adrenals take over hormone production. I tell patients to think of them as your B team. You want them to be in good shape for when they take over and are needed.

Although rare, **Addison's disease,** where the adrenal cortex fails to produce enough cortisol and aldosterone, can affect anyone at any age. Symptoms include severe fatigue, low blood pressure, darkening of the skin, weight loss, reduced appetite, low blood sugar, abdominal pains, irritability, muscle and joint pains, hair loss, and nausea, diarrhea, or vomiting. These patients are dependent on taking hydrocortisone for the rest of their lives. To meet criteria for Addison's, you must fail an adrenocorticotropic hormone (ACTH) stimulation test. This measures how well the adrenal glands respond to ACTH.

Cushing's syndrome is also uncommon. Think of it as the opposite of Addison's disease. In Cushing's there is overproduction of the hormone cortisol. Symptoms include weight gain around the midsection, in the face (moon face), and between the shoulders (buffalo hump), purple stretch marks on the skin, easy bruising, slow healing, acne, facial hair, and irregular menstrual cycles. Individuals with suspected Addison's or Cushing's should be assessed and managed by an endocrinologist.

ADRENAL FATIGUE

Stress is your body's biggest hormone hijacker. In times of stress, you may experience the fight-or-flight response. This is initiated by the sympathetic nervous system. The adrenals then secrete cortisol, adrenaline, epinephrine, and norepinephrine. However, this response can only last so long. I often see patients "crash and burn" following these times. Although I don't often see full-blown cases of Addison's disease, I very commonly see cases of adrenal stress, what some call **adrenal fatigue**.

Symptoms alone don't always dictate when patients are in a fight-or-flight response. It also shows on cortisol testing. On a twenty-four-hour urine test, cortisol metabolites can be high. However, a better test is a four- to five-point saliva test. With this test, individuals spit saliva into a collection tube multiple times throughout the day. Cortisol is supposed to be the highest in the morning and gently reduce throughout the day, being lowest at night to allow the individual to sleep. In times of stress, cortisol is often high even at night, inhibiting patients from sleeping well. Many patients have presented to me thinking they have Addison's, but then passed their ACTH stimulation test. However, they still could be experiencing adrenal stress—lower cortisol—and need support.

We can also test for neurotransmitters to see if the individual is producing a high or low amount of either *excitatory*, energizing neurotransmitters such as dopamine, norepinephrine, and epinephrine, or *inhibitory*, calming neurotransmitters such as serotonin, GABA, and taurine. If they are very anxious or having problems sleeping, they could be high in excitatory neurotransmitters or low in calming neurotransmitters. Once tested, we can then recommend various lifestyle changes and supplements to help balance the neurotransmitters. Remember, neurotransmitters are made in the gut, in the adrenals, and in the brain.

When the adrenals are stressed, they can't effectively help with sex or thyroid hormone production. Managing your stress is critical for optimal cortisol and neurotransmitter production. Your adrenals need "down time." They need recovery and healing time. Your body can't function well under continuous stress.

I too have experienced years of high stress with so much on my plate. My sympathetic nervous system was overworked and I was stuck in the fight-or-flight mode for too long, and as a result my body paid the price. I am now recovered, and know how to not let that happen again.

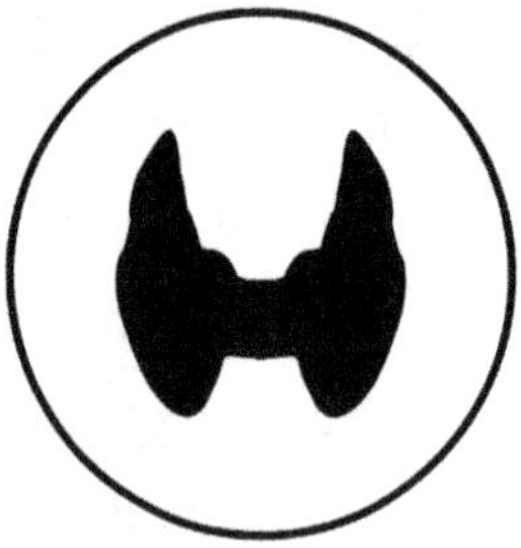

THYROID GLAND AND THYROID HORMONE PRODUCTION

The thyroid is a butterfly-shaped gland located in front of your trachea (windpipe) and just below the larynx (Adam's apple) in the neck. It has two lobes or halves. The main function of the thyroid gland is to regulate your metabolism, or your body's ability to break down food and convert it to energy. It is able to do this by making thyroid hormones from iodine taken from the blood. The pituitary gland and hypothalamus both control the thyroid. As David Brownstein writes: "Every single muscle, organ and cell in the body depends on adequate thyroid hormone levels for achieving and maintaining optimal functioning" (Brownstein 2002, 33).

The hypothalamus secretes thyrotropin-releasing hormones (TRH), which tells the pituitary to produce thyroid-stimulating hormones (TSH), which then tells the thyroid to start producing thyroid hormones. The two main thyroid hormones are tri-iodothyronine (T3) and thyroxine (T4). The thyroid also produces calcitonin, which helps to control blood calcium levels.

Hypothyroidism occurs when the levels of thyroid hormone are too low. Typically, individuals start to feel sluggish and feel their metabolism slowing as thyroid function declines. Symptoms of

hypothyroidism include fatigue, depression, weakness, dry hair and skin, hair loss, cold intolerance, constipation, memory fog, irregular menstrual cycles, low libido, muscle aches, and cramps. If left untreated, hypothyroidism can lead to heart failure and even coma.

Autoimmune conditions occur when the body attacks itself. **Hashimoto's thyroiditis** is a common autoimmune disease that occurs due to destruction of the thyroid gland. This damage leads to reduced thyroid function and lower thyroid hormone levels. It is the number one cause of hypothyroidism. Ninety percent of individuals with Hashimoto's have elevated thyroid peroxidase antibodies (TPOAb), and 80 percent have elevated thyroglobulin antibodies (TgAb).

Other causes of hypothyroidism include surgical removal of part of the thyroid gland due to goiters or nodules, and problems with the pituitary gland. If the pituitary doesn't send the proper signal to the thyroid, then the thyroid doesn't make the hormones.

Hyperthyroidism occurs when the level of thyroid hormones are too high. Symptoms include heat sensitivities, hyperactivity, increased appetite, palpitations, insomnia, nerve tingling, nervousness, menstrual irregularities, and weight loss.

I also commonly see an enlarged thyroid or bulge in the neck, also known as a **goiter**. This is typically caused by iodine deficiency. A goiter is sometimes a side effect of hyperthyroidism because of an overstimulated and inflamed thyroid. A goiter can also occur without the individual being hyperthyroid. Goiters can be treated by surgical removal or by radioactive iodine treatment, the goal being to destroy the part of the thyroid that is growing larger or producing too much thyroid hormone. In many cases after testing iodine levels, I've seen iodine help reduce goiters as well.

Unfortunately, sometimes the entire thyroid is destroyed (through treatment) and the patient becomes hypothyroid, and thus dependent on thyroid medication. As mentioned, Hashimoto's is an autoimmune hypothyroid condition. Likewise, **Graves' disease** is an autoimmune hyperthyroid condition. Patients with Graves' often have protruding eyes, goiters, a fast heart rate, and tingling sensations.

I often find thyroid nodules in my patients as well. It's estimated that half the population may have nodules, most of which are benign, and some of which can lead to cancer. If detected early, prognosis for thyroid cancer is good, and long-term survival rates are excellent. If you think you have an enlarged thyroid gland, have your medical provider palpate or feel it at your appointment. If abnormal, a diagnostic thyroid ultrasound can be ordered to determine if there are nodules, cysts, or enlargements.

There are several excellent books about the thyroid alone, including *Overcoming Thyroid Disorders,* by David Brownstein, MD, *Why Do I Still Have Thyroid Symptoms? When My Labs Are Normal,* by Datis Kharrazian, MD, and *Stop the Thyroid Madness,* by Janie A. Bowthorpe. Each of these books has its own Facebook group with excellent, updated information. *Hashimoto's Thyroiditis: Lifestyle Interventions for Finding and Treating the Root Cause*, by Izabella Wentz, MD, focuses specifically on Hashimoto's. Her approach, which she terms "DIG-AT-IT," encourages patients to get to the root cause of their Hashimoto's by exploring nutritional deficiencies, digestion issues, infections, food intolerances, and toxins—the same concepts I'm discussing in this book (Wentz 2013). Her book is the most comprehensive writing I have seen on Hashimoto's, and it is highly recommended reading. She also mentions many of the tests I discuss in this book.

SEX HORMONE TESTING

Testing should always be individualized based on what the patient is taking. Serum or blood levels are the best-accepted, FDA-cleared methods of testing. They are a reliable means for testing reproductive hormones and thyroid hormones. However, for women, they must be interpreted in the context of a period cycle. For instance, you may choose to test for FSH on day three of a woman's cycle, but not test progesterone until a week after ovulation around day nineteen or twenty. You would expect FSH to be low and the progesterone to be high at their respective times of testing in a young, cycling, fertile woman. I typically reserve blood testing for postmenopausal women whose hormones aren't fluctuating anymore, or for a fertility workup when patients can time the testing as advised.

Urine testing is the best and only way to detect phase 1 and 2 estrogen metabolites. You can run a six-hour test, but a twenty-four-hour or dried urine test for metabolites is better. I use Genova Diagnostics for twenty-four-hour urine testing, and Precision Analytical offers a dried urine test for a comprehensive hormone assessment (DUTCH) where you can see metabolites as well as the diurnal cortisol pattern not seen in a twenty-four-hour urine test. Meridian Valley also offers a comprehensive twenty-four-hour test.

Saliva testing is the best means to test cortisol. It is also great for fertility, because it allows visualization of hormone levels through the monthly cycle. It allows for assessment of fluctuations and variations from normal. This is one way to test hormones through the entire month while the patient logs their symptoms for premenstrual headaches or even headaches with ovulation. This is also a great way to identify if progesterone is dropping at the wrong time or if luteal phase defects exist.

How I choose to test patients' levels is also determined by what type of hormone replacement therapy the patient is taking. For instance, if the patient is taking oral estrogen or oral progesterone, I measure these with blood. If I want to see metabolites, those can be measured in the urine. If a patient has a family history of cancer, urine is the best test. I'll explain why when I discuss estrogen metabolism.

If patients are using injectable testosterone, serum levels are appropriate. If the patient is using a transdermal cream, these levels can be very difficult to monitor. Typically, these will skew saliva reference ranges very high. There is really no highly reliable test for topical hormone usage. I often use urine testing for patients using topical options. If you're using blood work, application time matters. Depending on when the patient applies the topical gel or cream in relation to when the labs are drawn, the test may capture a peak or a trough that should be taken into consideration with dosing changes.

If patients are using sublingual hormones, it's also important to know if you are capturing a peak or trough. For instance, if a patient takes a sublingual hormone three hours before he gets his blood drawn, you will likely see a peak. The level viewed is the highest it will be all day, since levels will drop the rest of the day. Sublingual hormones also skew saliva; therefore, a twenty-four-hour urine test is the best way to assess sublingual usage. However, with this test, it is best for the patient to allow the sublingual to dissolve, and then spit out the rest to avoid first-pass metabolism contamination. No hormone will be cleared through the gut or liver if it is not swallowed.

Precision Analytical lab has a very thorough testing matrix available on its website to help you determine the best means of testing.

I can't emphasize enough how very important it is to test levels and not treat patients based only on their symptoms. I had a woman with hot flashes come to me after seeing her OB/GYN, who put her on synthetic oral estrogen for hot flashes without testing any levels. Surprisingly, she did not have low estrogen at all. She was actually dangerously high in estrogen. She should never have been given estrogen. Once I tested her levels, we found that she needed progesterone and testosterone, which I gave her. Once I took her off the estrogen and helped her through an estrogen detox, her hot flashes resolved.

ESTROGEN METABOLISM

When discussing hormones, it's difficult not to bring up **cancer.** Breast cancer is the leading cause of cancer death among women. Health care providers' approach to breast cancer risk prevention is narrow, with few providers being familiar with available diagnostic tools such as genetic testing. Typically, the use of hormone replacement therapy is discouraged. The current, most logical treatment rationale for individuals with estrogen-related breast cancers is blocking estrogens using pharmaceuticals like Tamoxifen and aromatase inhibitors like Aromasin (Singh, Francis, and Michael 2011).

Interestingly, other researchers suspect that the most significant relationship between estrogens and cancer is not the level of estrogens themselves, but the metabolism by which the body detoxifies these estrogens. *That*, they believe, not the level of hormones in the body, impacts one's cancer risk. I tell my patients that it is important to identify not only their levels of hormones but also the means by which the body detoxifies or eliminates hormones. In other words, whether the patient is taking estrogen or not, we need to know where the hormones are going. We can check downstream metabolites to see how the liver is detoxifying hormones. This is what I wanted to study for my doctorate, and is where the urine hormone test comes in.

This next part gets a little complicated. Bear with me. Estrogens must be eliminated from the body after conversion to estrogenically inactive metabolites, which are eliminated in urine or stool. I use urine to test for these important metabolites. Roughly 80 percent of a woman's urinary metabolites are from estrone, and only 20 percent from estradiol and estriol. Postmenopausal women usually have more estrone to metabolize. The phase 1 metabolite (end product) of 2-hydroxylation, 2-hydroxyestrone, or 2-OHE1 is known as a "good" estrogen metabolite. It has a modest anti-estrogenic effect; thus, is less estrogenic (Zeligs et al. 2005). It is ideally high to help reduce cancer growth and inhibit angiogenesis (formation of new blood vessels). The phase 2 detoxification pathways include sulfation, glucuronidation, methylation, and a reaction with glutathionine. The phase 2 metabolite from 2-OHE1, 2-methoxyestrone (2-OmeE1) has been shown to have anticancerous effects and is ideal in high levels. The phase II metabolite from 4-OHE1, 4-methoxyestrone or 4-OmeE1 is also a non-cancerous metabolite (Zeligs et al. 2005). In comparison, a metabolite of 16 hydroxylation, 16α-hydroxyestrone, or 16α-OHE1, is an estrogen agonist having contrasting activity to 2-hydroxyestrone. It has a high affinity for estrogen receptors and is also known as the "bad" estrogen. Estrogen-sensitive tumors have tissue promoted by this metabolite. Having increased 16α-hydroxylation has been associated with higher cervical, endometrial, larynx, and breast cancer (Lord and Burdette 2006). 16α-hydroxyestrone is also ideally low, as high levels have been suspected to encourage tumor development. On the other hand, of the "bad" estrogen metabolites, ideally 4-hydroxyestrone levels are low, as high levels may react negatively with damaged DNA.

When discussing estrogen metabolites, remember that they can be tested: 2-OHE1 (2 hydroxy) and 4-OmeE1 (4 methoxy) are good. You want them at higher levels. While 4-OHE1 (4 hydroxy) and 16α-OHE1 (16α hydroxy) are bad—potentially carcinogenic—and you want them at lower levels. Many lab companies produce a 2/16 αhydroxyestrone ratio. If this ratio is low, the individual is at higher risk.

These metabolites may be easier to understand when the entire estrogen metabolism pathway is visualized.

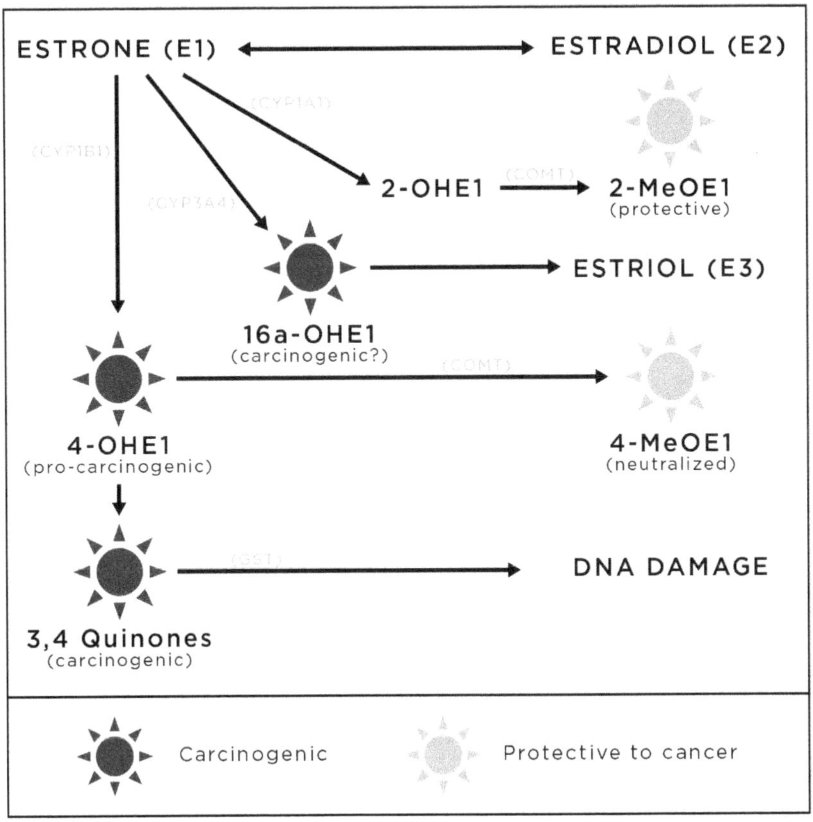

Remember COMT and GST from chapter 3? I included them within this graph to also show you how genetics also have an influence on estrogen metabolism.

TESTING THYROID HORMONE LEVELS

Hormones are essential to survival, and they decline as the body ages. How do you know if you have hormone imbalances? Test! In combination with symptoms, there are several labs that I order on every suspected thyroid patient. The good news is that low or high thyroid can be easily detected with blood work.

Thyroid-Stimulating Hormone

Thyroid-stimulating hormone (TSH) is a pituitary hormone, not a thyroid hormone. It is currently the most common screening test for thyroid disease; however, many clinicians feel it is not sensitive enough. Many of my patients have come to me with years of "normal" TSH levels. However, when I check functional free thyroxine (free T4) and free triiodothyronine (free T3) levels, these are low or barely in the reference range. As mentor Joseph Collins, ND, RN, once told me, TSH stands for "Too slow to help." By the time TSH is high, the patient has likely had low thyroid symptoms for a long time. I also have patients with subclinical hypothyroidism, where the TSH is rising but the free T4 and free T3 are still normal. Either way, TSH is not the best test. It is a feedback test from the brain, but think about it—that feedback mechanism isn't always perfect. If the feedback mechanism *is* intact, the higher the TSH, the more unsatisfied the body is with circulating thyroid hormone levels. It's screaming for help! I have also seen patients with a perfectly normal TSH yet low Free T4 and Free T3 levels.

Some believe the TSH range is too lax, considering that when the "normal" was created it included testing results of elderly patients, some with poor thyroid function. Regardless of what your local lab may use for a standard reference range, according to the American College of Endocrinology, TSH levels need to be between 0.3 and 3.0 uIU/mL. Many functional medicine providers, like me, aim to keep TSH below 2.

Thyroid Hormones

In order not to miss thyroid conditions, additional labs should be checked. Free T4 and free T3 are the body's main thyroid hormones. Both are made by the thyrocytes, the thyroid cell in the thyroid gland. Both are necessary to check. T4 is made from thyroglobulin joining up with four molecules of iodine. It is then taken up by the thyroid-binding protein. The liver then converts some T4 to T3 while other tissues convert the rest. However, many patients have poor T4-to-T3 conversion. Free T3 is three times as potent as T4. Your body only has T3 receptors. That means you could have very high T4 levels, but if they aren't converting to T3 and binding to receptors, their signal or message isn't getting sent. That high T4 level is essentially useless. Unfortunately, many of my patients do not convert their T4 to T3 well. This can be due to nutritional deficiencies in selenium or zinc, various medications such as birth control pills, steroids, beta blockers, cruciferous vegetables, soy, and toxins like alcohol, pesticides, mercury, and lead. It can also be due to elevated thyroid antibodies or adrenal stress.

That is also why patients could have normal TSH and normal or high free T4 and still be very symptomatic of low thyroid—because they aren't converting the free T4 to free T3. Also, some free T4 converts to reverse T3 (RT3). Think of your free T3 as the gas pedal on your metabolism. Reverse T3 is the brake. You don't want the brake to be on and gas pedal off. Reverse T3 is high in times of stress, surgery, trauma, and chronic illness.

According to Datis Kharrazian, interestingly, 20 percent of healthy thyroid functions depend on healthy gut flora, since thyroid hormones become inactive in the absence of healthy gut bacteria (Kharrazian 2010). Remember, gut health is the foundation in your Longevity Blueprint.

TSH fluctuates and can be checked at any time of day. However, hormones peak in the morning, making it the most appropriate time to check labs. If you are taking a medication containing T3 with a short half-life, and if your provider is trying to evaluate the effectiveness of that medication, you want it in your bloodstream at the time of testing. Therefore, if my patient takes their Nature-Throid at seven o'clock in the morning, a four o'clock afternoon lab draw would be useless. I require my patients take T3 and then come to the lab around the medication's approximate half-life, which is four to five hours after having taken it, around eleven o'clock in the morning in this case. Goals for free T4 and free T3 levels are the higher end of the normal range. I want my patients' free T3s around 3.5–4.0.

Thyroid Antibodies

Thyroid peroxidase (TPO) is an enzyme normally found in the thyroid gland. When the thyroid gland becomes inflamed, it can leak out this enzyme. The body then alerts an attack on the enzyme and creates antibodies against TPO in the blood, called thyroid peroxidase antibodies (Abs). Antithyroglobulin antibodies (Anti-TG) can be a sign of thyroid gland damage or destruction caused by the immune system. These are often also high in autoimmune diseases like Hashimoto's or Graves' disease. These antibodies can also fluctuate. I have seen this in lab testing where one day they show positive while another they are negative. This demonstrates how Hashimoto's can be missed.

Iodine

We've known for over fifty years how iodine deficiency can lead to goiters as well as mental retardation. Populations deficient in iodine can have devastating health consequences. T4 is made from a backbone of the amino acid tyrosine with four iodine molecules. T3 has three iodine molecules. Your thyroid won't function well without optimal iodine.

It's believed that people are now becoming iodine deficient due to being dominant in the halogen bromide. Halogens levels in our bodies are controlled by a mechanism called "competitive inhibition" (Farrow 2013, 67), which means they all compete for binding sites on the same receptors. Halogens include bromine, chlorine, fluorine, and astatine.

Chloride and fluoride can also cause endocrine problems by shoving out iodine. Don't take a long, hot shower without the vent or door open, as you can literally expose yourself to chlorine gas. Fluoride is in toothpaste and many dental treatment options. Ever notice the warning on your toothpaste tube: "If swallowed, please call poison control"? Fluoride is surprisingly found in many pharmaceutical drugs. Symptoms of toxicity include nausea, vomiting, diarrhea, abdominal pain, excessive salivation, and potentially neurological damage.

Human exposure to the anti-iodine, bromide, has increased, and some believe that, like the aforementioned halogens, it dominates receptor sites, shoving out the important iodine. In the 1970s, bromide was added to flour as a food fortifier while iodine was removed (Farrow 2013). It's now found in flame retardants, rugs, cars, mattresses, upholstery, hair dye, electronics, asthma medications, hot tub cleaners, and even pajamas, as the documentary *Stink* mentions. Even beverages, such as Mountain Dew, contain brominated vegetable oil.

There are currently two ways to test for low iodine. The skin patch test isn't the best available testing option, because your body could be dehydrated the day you test. Also, even if your skin does or doesn't need iodine that day, that's not necessarily reflective of how much your other organs, such as ovaries, may need. A better test is the iodine loading test, where the individual takes a high-dose iodine pill of 50 mg and then collects his or her urine over twenty-four hours. The more iodine excreted, the less deficient the body is. The less excreted (meaning the more the body soaks up) the more deficient the body is. If your body is already saturated with iodine, you urinate more of it.

If found to be low, supplementing can help. Lynne Farrow discusses in her book, *The Iodine Crisis: What You Don't Know About Iodine Can Wreck Your Life,* how iodine supplementation isn't a fad (Farrow 2013). In fact, iodine has been used as early as the 1820s, and was used well into the 1940s as a staple in medicine. The recommended daily allowance for iodine was calculated only on the amount the thyroid needs to avoid goiter, not on the amount the rest of the organs in the body need.

You'd have to consume four pounds of ocean fish daily to obtain the needed amounts of iodine, and you'd likely be subjecting yourself to loads of toxic mercury in the meantime. The Fukushima Japanese nuclear reactor explosion contaminated much of the world's seaweed, as have the various oil spills in the United States. Seaweed also may contain arsenic and heavy metals. Plus, you never know exactly how much iodine you will be getting in kelp consumption. And no, you can't get enough iodine from iodized table salt. By the time the iodized salt gets to the store, half the initial iodine content has been lost (vaporized), and only 10 percent of the iodine is absorbable. Plus, that is a bad combination anyway, as sodium chloride contains chloride, another halogen competing for binding sites. Also, cooking destroys iodine.

After completing the iodine loading test, a provider trained in functional medicine can help you determine the best dose for you. Iodine can be taken in capsule or liquid form. Two drops of Lugol's 5 percent solution equals 12.5 mg of an Iodoral tablet. I typically start patients (who are confirmed low through testing) on one drop or 6.25 mg and see how they tolerate that before slowly working up on dose. Building up the dose gradually will help to reduce side effects. The solution can stain clothes. A thick paste of vitamin C powder and water can help remove the stains. How long do you need to supplement? As long as you are exposed to halogens!

Controversy does exist over whether or not individuals with elevated thyroid antibodies should take iodine. Some believe iodine will help, while others believe giving iodine is like throwing gasoline onto an autoimmune fire. The theory here is that if iodine stimulates production of thyroid peroxidase enzyme, it could also fuel the TPO Abs flaring up the autoimmune condition. Drs. Jan Wolff and Israel Lyon Chaikoff first started the fear—now known as the Wolff-Chaikoff effect—that iodine was dangerous based on one study from 1948 that could never be replicated (Farrow 2013). Guy Abraham, MD, questioned this and eventually proved that iodine wasn't in fact dangerous (Farrow 2013). If my patients have been tested and need iodine, I give it, while monitoring thyroid antibody levels to verify they aren't on the rise.

Many individuals are concerned about the goitrogenic or thyroid-blocking effects of cruciferous vegetables. You won't experience this if you take iodine (Farrow 2013). However, when taking iodine, it can "chase bromine off its seats on the receptors," causing short-term bromide toxicity (Farrow 2013, 81). So, if you take iodine and feel sick, these side effects are likely due to iodine detoxing bromide faster than your kidneys and liver can handle them. The toxins can enter the bloodstream, thyroid, and brain, causing a variety of side effects. Some patients even feel sedated. You can develop headaches, fatigue, and a runny nose.

Saltwater helps to catch toxins like bromide and flushes them out of your system. The *salt-loading protocol* can be used in these instances to help reduce those negative symptoms. For this protocol, take one-fourth to one-half teaspoon of unrefined sea salt dissolved in one-half cup of water, followed by twelve to sixteen ounces of water. Repeat in thirty minutes, if needed. As always, discuss with your provider before trying the protocol, especially if you have other chronic health conditions. Only use unbleached, unprocessed, unrefined salt, free of any anticaking agents. If you continue to experience these symptoms, you can try pulse dosing to help remedy the detox symptoms. Pulse dosing means stopping the iodine but continuing salt loading for forty-eight hours to flush toxins out. Then try the iodine again at a lower dose.

David Brownstein discusses in his book, *Iodine: Why You Need It and Why You Can't Live Without It*, how protective iodine is for the thyroid against oxidative damage (Brownstein 2002). For further reading on iodine, consider reading *The Iodine Crisis: What You Don't Know About Iodine Can Wreck Your Life*, by Lynne Farrow.

Ferritin

Ferritin is a blood protein that contains iron. If your ferritin test reveals that your level is low, you could have iron deficiency anemia even if your iron level is normal. I tell patients to think of your ferritin as your pantry stocked with soup cans. Your body will rob "Peter to pay Paul," so it will use up all of what's in your pantry to make its iron in the kitchen look good, all the while depleting its ferritin. You must work to stock your ferritin "pantry" full of iron. For proper thyroid function, you must have optimal ferritin levels. Ferritin is required for utilization of T3. Additionally, many women who have optimized thyroid hormone levels but are still losing hair have low ferritin. Optimal ferritin levels for hair regrowth are >70 (Wentz 2013).

Thyroglobulin

A thyroglobulin tumor marker can be ordered if thyroid cancer is suspected. In these cases, it will be likely high. These levels should be undetectable or very low after the surgical removal of the thyroid and after radioactive iodine treatments. If they are not reduced, it can indicate cancerous residual tissue is still present.

According to the American Association of Clinical Endocrinologists, twenty-seven million Americans have thyroid dysfunction, and thirteen million go undiagnosed (Gaitonde, Rowley, and Sweeney 2012). I believe this may be due to lack of provider understanding about how important it is to check comprehensive levels.

INTERPRETING HORMONE LABS

In addition to being well balanced, hormones should also be optimized. No one wants to be the patient with very high estrogen and without any protective progesterone onboard. However, you also don't want all your hormones to be balanced but all low.

I calculate a percentage for certain lab values for my patients. Then I draw these percentages on a bell-shaped curve. I explain to the patient what percentage they are functioning at. For instance, if you were graded on a test, would you want to score 10-15 percent? Of course not, you should at least want to be over the 50th percentile, if not the 80th. You want to pass, after all. If you only scored 75 percent on a test, you barely passed. Do you want your T3, your gas pedal, operating at 20 percent or at 80 percent?

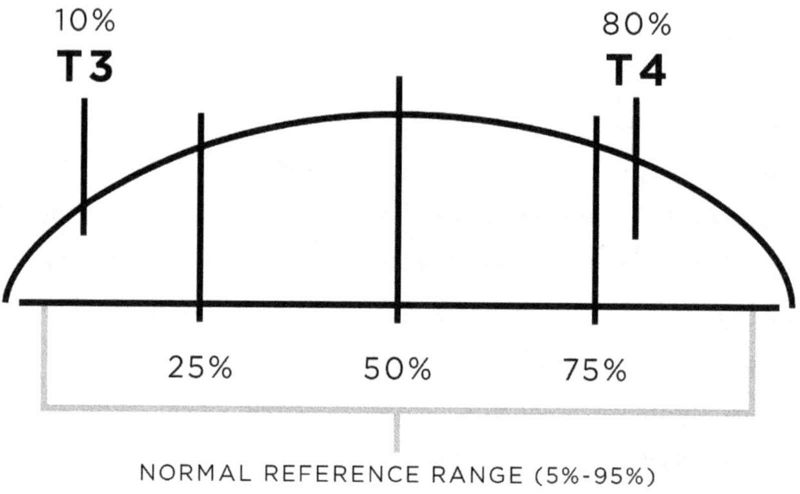

Functional medicine providers interpret labs differently than conventional providers. Your conventional provider may think your thyroid or hormone levels are in the normal range even if they are only at the 4th percentile!

Also, if you haven't had your hormone levels tested every few years, you won't know how much of a decline you are experiencing. For instance, if your levels dropped from the 85th percentile to the

30th, that is a significant decline and may accompany many negative symptoms. Yet you may still be considered in the "normal" reference range.

So how do we improve endocrine gland function and hormone production? First, we collect a thorough patient history to better understand the symptoms the patient is experiencing. Then, we determine the best means to test labs. Once we have the results, then we must determine how best to improve hormone function.

In *What You Must Know About Women's Hormones,* Pam Smith, MD, emphasizes the importance of removing any stressors that could compromise hormone production, and fixing nutritional deficiencies (Smith 2008). Our hormone pathways are dependent on it.

I once had a female patient who was suffering with menopausal symptoms. All I did was place her on two fish oil supplements and a multivitamin per day, and her hot flashes entirely resolved. This was a classic case of nutritional deficiencies not allowing hormone pathways to work as they should. Obviously, not every case is this easy; however, each symptomatic patient should absolutely have a nutritional deficiency test while concurrently being started on natural hormone replacement therapy.

In *Sexy Forever: How To Fight Fat After Forty*, Suzanne Somers discusses how important it is to detox. Toxins slow down metabolism and hormone production, and can lead to weight gain. A great first step to lose weight is to undergo a detox program. Detoxing can help to improve your sex hormone production.

We lastly must reduce stress on the adrenals so that they can help with thyroid and sex hormone production.

NUTRACEUTICAL SUPPLEMENTS FOR THE ADRENALS

Remember, if the adrenals are under stress, they can't help to produce sex and thyroid hormone levels. This will also result in poor T4-to-T3 conversion. Therefore, many of my hormone patients are placed on herbal adaptogenic support to help the body adapt to stress better.

The top studied adaptogenic herbs that help the body adapt to stress are Rhodiola, Eleutherococcus senticosus, Schisandra, and Ashwagandha. ***Rhodiola rosea*** can help to support the nervous system, mood, mental clarity, work performance, and the sleep cycle. It can also help to preserve levels of neurotransmitters such as serotonin, dopamine, and norepinephrine. ***Eleutherococcus senticosus*** has been used for memory and endurance. It is helpful for improving energy levels, specifically in endurance athletes. ***Schisandra chinensis*** can help with mental clarity, stress response, and emotional well-being. It can support increased blood flow through the body as well. ***Ashwaganda*** is helpful for memory, mood, energy, and endurance. It helps to improve cortisol levels and also has a thyroid hormone balancing effect.

Various adrenal support formulations exist. Some individuals have high cortisol and need calming down. For these individuals, I use an adaptogen blend with the calming amino acid L-theanine (mentioned in chapter 4), and an phosphatidyl serine—a phospholipid—both of which help reduce the half-life of cortisol. This Longevity Blueprint (LB) product is called Adrenal Calm. Other individuals need more stimulation. For these individuals, I recommend adrenal support containing an adrenal glandular concentrate from bovine (cow). The theory behind glandular therapy is that similar organ extracts from animals may support the same organ within humans by stimulating their activity. This LB product is called Adrenal Drive. We also carry a straight Herbal Adrenal Complex.

I also use hydrocortisone replacement, but only when absolutely necessary. I've had patients who didn't fail the ACTH stimulation test, yet who still had very low cortisol, and could barely function through the day; these patients greatly benefited from a modest dose of hydrocortisone, 5 to 20 mg daily. This replacement is described in detail in the book *Safe Uses of Cortisol*, by William McK. Jefferies, MD. I use this only after I've tried the patient on an adrenal glandular first.

Salt is essential for every cell in the body. It is extremely important for the adrenal glands. As mentioned previously, I recommend my hormone patients also add high-quality sea salt to their meals daily.

Licorice root extract is often added to herbal adrenal formulations. It helps prevent low blood pressure, and helps to extend the half-life of cortisol. It should only be taken in small doses to help maintain cortisol levels.

NUTRACEUTICAL SUPPLEMENTS FOR SEX HORMONE PRODUCTION

Herbs are great for younger women. At my practice, I use various herbal formulations created by a naturopathic doctor and friend, Dr. Joseph Collins. These are available for you to view at www.yourlongevityblueprint.com. Herbs can take weeks to months for full effect. However, they can be very effective.

EstroMend™ is an herbal formulation with a synergistic blend of the top estrogen-enhancing herbs such as red clover, isoflavones, and black cohosh. ProgestoMend™ is an herbal formulation that includes a synergistic blend of vitex, passionflower, and paeonae, to name a few. TestoGain™ is the herbal formulation designed to increase testosterone and includes herbs such as horny goatweed and tribulus. On occasion, for hormone imbalances like polycystic ovarian syndrome when women have high levels of androgens, we can use herbs like those found in TestoQuench™ for women to reduce the androgens. In men with high estrogen, we can use herbs like those found in EstroQuench™ to reduce estrogens.

NUTRACEUTICAL SUPPLEMENTS FOR HORMONE METABOLISM

Amongst conventional providers, there is an alarming lack of knowledge regarding the availability to test estrogen metabolism as well as nutritional interventions to facilitate healthy estrogen metabolism and ultimately decrease breast cancer risk.

Specifically, if the 2/16α-hydroxyestrone ratio is low, and disease risk high, providers can encourage nutritional interventions to raise this ratio, decreasing a patient's risk profile. As consistently found in the literature, 300 mg DIM is recommended for individuals with 2/16 ratios that are not within goal. DIM is the active indole molecule from cruciferous vegetables. If, after testing, the 4-hydroxyestrone is elevated, antioxidants like N-acetylcysteine and resveratrol should be recommended. If the methoxyestrogens are low, methylating cofactors should be given to include SAM-e, B6, 5MTHF, B12, DMG, and TMG. The previously recommended combination of nutrients may effectively support the preferred estrogen detoxification pathways over the risk-inducing pathways. This can potentially be profoundly significant for prevention of estrogen-related cancers such as estrogen-receptor-positive breast cancer. I put all my patients on hormones with LB DIM and LB Methyl B Complex as an extra insurance plan.

NUTRACEUTICAL SUPPLEMENTS FOR THYROID

Several herbs can help with thyroid hormone production, including guggulipid, bacopa, ashwagandha, hops, coleus forskohli, sage, and rosemary.

For enhancing thyroid function, I typically recommend 200 mcg selenium to my thyroid patients. Selenium not only helps convert T4 to T3, it can also help reduce thyroid peroxidase antibodies (Gärtner et al. 2002). Brazil nuts are high in selenium. Many of my patients try to eat a few of these daily.

I also recommend various doses of iodine, depending on the results of my patient's iodine tests. The amino acid tyrosine is often recommended at 500 mg twice daily. Tyrosine is an integral part of thyroid hormone production together with iodine. Glutathione is a powerful antioxidant that can help to protect the thyroid against oxidative stress and damage. This is very important for autoimmune cases.

Taking natural anti-inflammatories is also critical, especially with the presence of autoimmune diseases. The most common anti-inflammatories I recommend are turmeric and omega-3s from fish oil. My favorite LB herbal thyroid health product is Thyroid Complex.

I also recommend assessing for specific nutritional deficiencies, which are discussed in chapter 4, since many nutrients can influence thyroid function.

The hallmark dietary change for individuals with autoimmune thyroid conditions is a gluten-free diet, since these patients are at a significantly higher risk for celiac disease. Gluten is the protein found in wheat, barley, rye, and contaminated oats. Molecular mimicry, also discussed in chapter 1, is a fairly new theory that explains how our immune system may attack healthy cells. The molecular structure of gluten resembles the thyroid peroxidase enzyme. Thus eating gluten could also fuel an autoimmune fire and should be avoided. Additionally, these patients should be tested for other food sensitivities, as mentioned in chapter 1, that can also be their personal triggers to inflammation.

I have seen thyroid antibody levels drop tremendously in compliant patients who have removed their inflammatory trigger foods like gluten. The end result is improved thyroid function.

HORMONE REPLACEMENT THERAPY

I specialize in natural hormone replacement therapy (NHRT). Hormone replacement therapy is not considered a one-size-fits-all approach. Not every single woman with, for instance, hot flashes, —regardless of her age, weight, or hysterectomy status—should be given the exact same dose of oral Premarin. That's not respecting each woman's biochemical individuality. Every patient in our clinic is treated individually. Everyone first has hormone testing, and then we determine the best way to achieve the optimal hormone balance for that patient.

I've had patients come to me from several other hormone clinics where they were started on hormones and their levels were never assessed again. I cannot emphasize the importance of this enough. The patient's need for hormones could increase or decrease dependent on their current hormone function and stress status, even if they are developing a bit of dermal fatigue or receptor resistance with topical use. This needs to be assessed on an annual basis and when patients are feeling symptomatic.

Comparing Natural to Synthetic Hormones

Commonly, when hormone replacement therapy is discussed, the first question that I am asked is, "Don't hormones cause cancer?" No, hormones do not cause cancer. If they did, we would see a bunch of twenty-year-olds walking around with cancer and a bunch of ninety-year-olds very cancer-free—and that is simply not something you see. Ninety-year-olds have a greater risk for cancer and the lowest level of hormones, and twenty-year-olds have a reduced risk for cancer and the highest levels of hormones.

However, the biggest point of contention and confusion is the type of hormones that are being given, as well as the dose and the route of administration.

It's difficult to discuss hormones without referencing the Women's Health Initiative trial. This study scared patients and providers away from using hormones. In the trial, synthetic estrogen and synthetic progestins were used. The estrogen used was Premarin, which comes from pregnant mares' urine. There's nothing natural about taking horse urine. Thus, estrogen was primarily estrone (the more dangerous of the estrogens). Also, this estrogen was given by mouth. The study showed:

- 41 percent increase in stroke
- 29 percent increase in heart attacks
- 26 percent increase in breast cancer
- Twice the rate of blood clots
- 76 percent increase in Alzheimer's and dementia

Needless to say, there weren't many prescriptions given for synthetic hormones after the study was published. Interestingly, the number one prescribed drug in America after the Women's Health Initiative study became Prozac, an antidepressant (Wehrwein 2011).

In comparison, these side effects have not been seen in studies where natural hormones were used. In fact, studies using natural hormones show reduced cancer risk, reduced cardiovascular disease, and reduced Alzheimer's risk. Deborah Moskowitz reviewed the safety of bioidentical hormones in 2006. She concluded that bioidentical hormones have demonstrated effectiveness and safety and recommends their use over synthetic. I agree with Moskowitz. Sadly, many individuals and medical providers do *not* differentiate natural from synthetic, and assume they both have the same risks, when they do not.

NATURAL PROGESTERONE VS. SYNTHETIC MEDROXYPROGESTERONE ACETATE (MDPA)

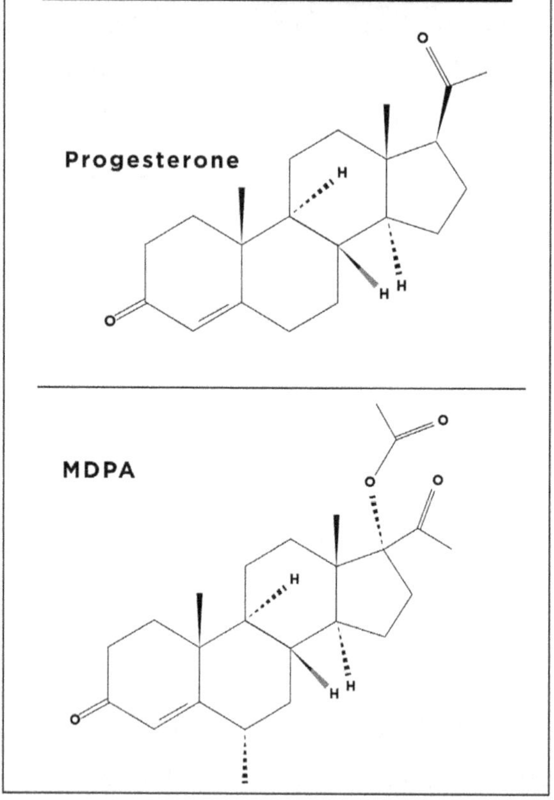

The major difference between synthetic and natural is the chemical structure. The chemical structure of medroxyprogesterone acetate (MDPA), a populate synthetic progestin, and the chemical structure of natural progesterone show obvious differences. MDPA is more difficult for your body to recognize and use, since it doesn't bind to progesterone receptors appropriately. It only binds partially and thus causes more side effects. Natural progesterone is biologically identical to the progesterone your body makes and thus binds appropriately and doesn't cause the side effects of the synthetics. The same is true for synthetic estrogen and testosterone versus natural. Since we're comparing our endocrine system to the heating/cooling system in our home, think about your furnace filters. The filter has to fit for it to serve a purpose and actually work. The same is true with hormones—the synthetics won't fit as well as the natural hormones will.

NATURAL TESTOSTERONE VS. SYNTHETICS

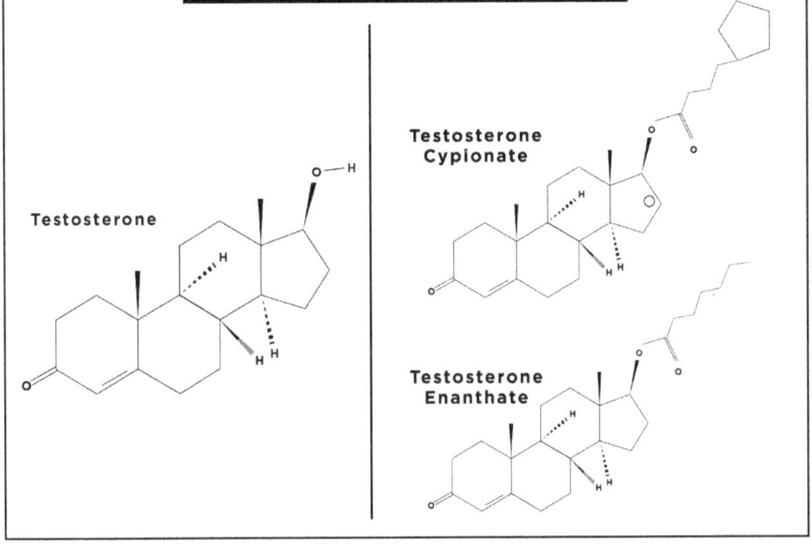

Through my experiences over the years, I've had several patients not tolerate synthetic hormones well at all. For instance, I had a middle-aged male patient who had terrible anxiety from synthetic testosterone, but he tolerated the natural version well. In fact, he felt amazing on the natural and received all the benefits he had hoped to receive from synthetic but never did. Interestingly, he is a medical doctor and his eyes were opened through this process with his health. His skepticism for natural hormones was erased and he now shares what he has learned with others.

Delivery Methods for Hormones

The most common way that I prescribe progesterone to menopausal woman is in a **capsule** form. This is a bioidentical natural progesterone option typically compounded by a compounding pharmacy. Micronized progesterone is also available at some commercial pharmacies; however, since this medication is not compounded, the dose can vary by 30 percent. Oftentimes, commercially available medications contain lactose or other allergens and dyes that many of my patients cannot tolerate. For patients with problems sleeping, when compounding, I can specify the progesterone to be a fast-acting or sustained release (SR) version.

I also prescribe **sublingual (SL)** or under-the-tongue options for women who do not want to take progesterone by mouth because they have experienced gas or bloating when taking it. This could have been from lactose in the capsule. However, SL is also my favorite way to give progesterone to a cycling woman, as she can taper her dose up and down through the last two weeks of her cycle, also known as the luteal phase. We do this to mimic what should be happening with natural progesterone rise and decline through the month.

Topical creams and gels are available and I prescribe these, although not frequently since I have not found them to be nearly as effective as sublingual or oral versions. These are, however, great for patients with major sensitivities who can't tolerate the stronger versions.

Progesterone is typically given at night, because it is so calming and can help with sleep. I have seen it lower blood pressure, so for women who already have very low blood pressure, I encourage them to monitor this.

Many gynecologists do not feel the need to give women progesterone when they are taking estradiol, specifically if they do *not* have a uterus. The theory is that if the woman does not have a uterus, she does not need to take progesterone to protect her from the estrogen. However, just because she does not have a uterus anymore does not mean her remaining breasts do not need protection. As mentioned, estrogen is proliferative, meaning it causes growth of tissues and causes growth of the endometrial lining. Progesterone is anti-proliferative, or antigrowth. It helps control the growth that estrogen could cause. I've been trained that every woman on estrogen needs progesterone. However, again, the best way to confirm need is to test hormone levels. Progesterone usually falls long before estradiol does.

I prefer to never give estradiol by mouth, since oral estrogen was what was used in the Women's Health Initiative. Instead, I use SL estradiol and estriol. I never give estrone. I also prescribe vaginal estradiol, but more commonly vaginal estriol, specifically for vaginal dryness and incontinence. With the exception of using vaginal estrogen only, for most occurrences, if I prescribe women estradiol I also give progesterone.

For years I prescribed topical testosterone to my patients. Many of my patients complained about how the topical smelled, that didn't dry well, and that it didn't provide the relief they had hoped for. I switched many of these patients over to SL therapy, which was much more effective. However, this created a peak-and-trough effect. Hours after taking it, the testosterone level would peak and then wear off throughout the day, leaving some patients moody. I also found that much of the testosterone would convert to estrogens, leaving patients with lower-than-expected testosterone levels.

I then decided to become certified in BioTE hormone **pellet therapy**. I quickly learned this was the safest, most effective way for my patients to achieve optimal testosterone levels. Both estradiol and testosterone can be given in this pellet form. Pellets are plant based, typically from wild yams. The compounded hormone powder is pressed in a dye, converting it to the shape of a pellet or grain of rice. In the office, after a small amount of an anesthetic like lidocaine is injected, it is then inserted into the subcutaneous (fatty) tissue in the upper buttocks.

The great benefit is that they are released over three to six months' time. They are released based on cardiac output. When you are sleeping, your body doesn't need a high level of testosterone. When you are exercising, your heart rate rises and blood flows past the pellet, bringing that testosterone into the bloodstream for you to use. When summertime is here and my active bike riding patients participate in Iowa's weeklong Ragbrai ride across the state, they will use more of their pellets that week than any other week of the year.

Interestingly, pellets are the oldest studied form of hormone replacement therapy, dating back to 1939 (Mishell 1941). They have been considered safe and effective since that time. Pellets do not increase risk for blood clots like other forms can. They are also extremely convenient, reducing the need to take a daily pill, SL troche, or cream, or to apply a patch every few days. The form avoids the fluctuations seen with all other forms of hormone replacement therapy. The release of pellets mimics the body's natural release of estradiol and testosterone.

Synthetic **injectable** testosterone is metabolized in the liver and can increase risk of heart diseases and, some believe, cancer. In contrast, bioidentical or natural testosterone is protective of the heart and lowers risk of advanced prostate cancer. In contrast, subcutaneous hormone pellets are not cleared through the liver. They are excreted in kidneys.

PERTAINING TO MALES

An exciting study, the *Mayo Clinical 2016 Consensus Recommendation* authored by Abraham Morgentaler, the Harvard urologist who taught in my fellowship program, states, "There is no scientific basis for any age specific recommendations against the use of testosterone therapy in men ... The evidence does not support increased risks of cardiovascular events with T therapy ... The evidence does not support increased risk for prostate cancer with T therapy" (Morgentaler 2016).

Another study, coauthored by Dr. Morgentaler, explains, "Contrary to traditional teaching, high endogenous serum testosterone does not increase the risk of prostate cancer, and low serum testosterone does not protect against prostate cancer" (Morgentaler 2016). Another study by Morgentaler and Traish in 2009 explains the saturation point: "Prostate growth is exquisitely sensitive to variations in androgen concentrations at very low concentrations, but becomes insensitive to changes in androgen concentrations at higher levels" (Morgentaler and Traish 2009). He explains that the prostate becomes saturated with androgens like testosterone at very low levels. Thus, increasing a man's level from 300 to 900 with hormone replacement therapy shouldn't increase any risk to his prostate, since it was already saturated with testosterone prior to the replacement therapy.

Natural testosterone pellets provide protection to the brain, heart, bones, joints, breast, and prostate. If you'd like to read more about hormone pellet therapy, consider reading *Age Healthier Live Happier,* by Gary Donovitz, MD, and visit www.BioTEmedical.com.

Fat cells secrete an enzyme called aromatase. Testosterone can aromatize, meaning it can convert to estrogen through that enzyme. Many of my younger male patients do not even need testosterone replacement; they need to reduce their estrogens. They need aromatase inhibitors. This is why it is so important to check all the sex hormones comprehensively. If needed, natural hormones can be given safely and effectively. I do recommend both DIM and EstroQuench™ in my male patients to help keep estrogens down.

THYROID REPLACEMENT THERAPY

Conventional thyroid replacement for hypothyroidism is T4 only. These options include synthroid, levothyroxine, levoxyl, and levothroid. They typically contain corn, and sometimes gluten and lactose. For some individuals, these drug options are a good fit, but for others they are not. More commonly, patients come to me having failed conventional T4-only replacement and wanting a product that is hypoallergenic. They have taken synthroid without symptom relief. They have poor T4-to-T3 conversion, or they may have a sensitivity to an ingredient in the T4-only options. They want instead to take a more natural, bioidentical thyroid replacement, a desiccated porcein (pig) option. Although this sounds odd, this is the closest version to our own thyroid hormone that is available. These desiccated options include Armour thyroid, Naturethroid, NP Thyroid, and Westhroid Pure (WP thyroid). They are still only given by prescription. Armour thyroid is an older option. I've been prescribing newer versions like Naturethroid or WP, since these are gluten-free versions. Cytomel is a widely used synthetic form of T3. However, it only comes in two doses: 5 mcg, which I prescribe, and 25 mcg, which is far too high a dose for many of my patients. If a patient is given too much thyroid replacement, they can experience symptoms of hyperthyroidism: palpitations, jitteriness, and insomnia. The dose should then be adjusted down.

Several studies have shown patients given T4 and T3 in combination feel better than patients given T4 only. These patients report improved mood and brain function (Bunevicius et al. 1999). Some providers are afraid that using natural desiccated thyroid will cause hyperthyroidism and lead to cardiac arrhythmias and bone loss. Research shows it does not. A study by Tammas Kelly, Lawerence Denmark, and Daniel Lieberman regarding use of desiccated thyroid replacement concluded that, "high circulating levels of thyroid hormone is not the cause of the sequela of hyperthyroidism. The reluctance to using high dose thyroid is unwarranted" (Kelly, Denmark, and Lieberman 2016).

If a provider is concerned, they should closely monitor their patients. I ask each patient on desiccated thyroid if they are experiencing any signs or symptoms of hyperthyroidism. Kelly, Denmark, and Lieberman also discuss the lack of evidence that exogenous desiccated thyroid causes osteoporosis or cardiac abnormalities (Kelly, Denmark, and Lieberman 2016).

I've had patients with pig allergies or religious beliefs against consuming pork products. For these cases, thyroid hormones T4 and T3 can also be compounded by a compounding pharmacist. This allows any allergens to be removed from the product. It is also one way to refine T4/T3 dosing for each patient. One of the beauties of compounding is the ability to have the pharmacist formulate a sustained release (SR) version that is released throughout the day and doesn't peak and drop so quickly, causing fewer side effects.

COMPOUNDING

From my experience, compounding pharmacists can be extremely helpful in finding tolerable options, especially for patients with multiple allergies or sensitivities. This is even important when compounding hormones. Many patients can't tolerate the base of the sublingual troches, and the pharmacies have to make them a special preparation.

It can be very difficult to find a great compounding pharmacy. I've been blessed to work with several, some in my city and others out of town. Hopefully, the provider prescribing the compound for you will be familiar with a great pharmacy near you. If not, here are some things to consider.

Use compounding pharmacies that have received Professional Compounding Centers of America (PCCA) certification. The Pharmacy Compounding Accreditation Board (PCAB) is a nonprofit organization that provides a voluntary accreditation program for compounding pharmacies nationwide. Ask if your compounding pharmacy is PCAB accredited. Also ask if the employed pharmacists have been to the intense compounding training provided by Professional Compounding Centers of America (PCCA). Ask if the compounding pharmacy performs batch testing on their compounded prescriptions. This will prove the purity and potency of the compounded medications. Does the pharmacy have a quality assurance program? Also, if you can't find a pharmacy in your state to compound your needed medication, make sure the pharmacy you find out of state is licensed to ship to your state. You can even ask if the pharmacy purchases US pharmaceutical grade (USP) chemicals from FDA registered suppliers. Also consider, as a patient of a compounding pharmacy, do you feel you were provided appropriate education on your medication?

CONCLUSION

Gina is a great example of patients we commonly see that need the Longevity Blueprint. She also had irritable bowel syndrome. We tested her for food sensitivities and properly assessed her hormones. She needed more than she had been given. It was discovered that her T4 wasn't converting to T3. She was switched off synthroid and onto Naturethroid, containing T3. She also needed progesterone, testosterone, and a safer route to take estradiol. She had been taking synthetic estrogen for years. We switched her from oral Premarin to estradiol pellets with the addition of testosterone. She likely had low progesterone since her twenties, since low progesterone could have caused the heavy bleeding and contributed to the endometriosis she had the hysterectomy for. I placed her on sustained release oral compounded progesterone at night, and we drastically changed her eating habits. In just two years, her bone density had normalized. She had totally transformed.

Cynthia needed a provider to listen to her health history, to discover when all of her "mental health" symptoms started (after a major stressor in her life, a divorce). Her hormone levels were terribly low. She required a steady, stable dosing of estrogen, testosterone in pellets, and SL progesterone daily. Her psychiatrists were amazed at her transformation. She is now off all her antipsychotic medications. She is happily remarried and now able to enjoy her husband and grandchildren. She truly has her life back.

You can read her and other patients' full testimonies on www.ihhclinic.com. You will see how the above women believe 100 percent that hormones changed their lives, and they are so thankful to have found a provider who would help them. Sadly, it took these women years to find a provider willing to assess and treat their hormones.

Can you imagine if you couldn't find a technician to help you with the heating and cooling system in your house for a decade?

Over the years, I've had several patients see an endocrinologist either before they came to see me or while they were seeing me. Many endocrinologists have not been taught anything outside of mainstream medicine. Many of them are not comfortable using desiccated thyroid or T3 therapy. Additionally, in my area of the country, it has been very difficult to find other conventional specialists who are willing to work with an integrative or functional provider who has been trained in using hormones like T3 or testosterone replacement therapy. These hormones are life-changing for some patients, and when providers aren't willing to learn about them and use them, patients are often left unassisted and feeling that their life is withering away without quality. They feel abandoned, frustrated, and hopeless.

Patients have shared with us the success of a saved marriage because of hormone optimization. They have shared with us how significant their transformations have been, how their lives have often been saved. We are incredibly thankful for the opportunity to help them along their hormone journeys.

Rather than detecting low testosterone at the age of fifty, I prefer all my patients have hormone levels checked in their twenties, thirties, and forties so that we can detect these subtle changes before hormone levels have eventually declined. This is true prevention.

Patients who are extremely compliant, who change their diets, minimize their stressors, and remove all toxins, are not as much in need of hormone replacement therapy as those who have ongoing stressors and are not willing to change their lifestyle.

Referring back to the fireman-versus-carpenter approach, we absolutely need trained specialists like urologists to test for and remove prostate cancer, and endocrinologists to test for and remove thyroid cancers. However, after having these fires removed, many patients are left, sadly, with *no* education on how to prevent future fires. I have never had a patient return to me stating that their conventionally trained provider discussed with them the importance of reducing endocrine-disrupting chemicals or toxins in their lives to prevent future cancers. Patients are left to conduct their research at home online, educating themselves on their journey to prevent future fires and cancer for themselves and future generations. We are here to help optimize hormones and help prevent future fires. Remember, if all you do is get your hormones balanced, you will be in better shape, but know that there is more to your Longevity Blueprint.

Longevity Blueprint Nutraceutical Products

Here are my favorite LB nutrients.

- Iodine 3
- Thyroid Complex
- Herbal Adrenal Complex
- Adrenal Drive
- Adrenal Calm
- DIM
- MethylB Complex

Chapter 6 Resources

A4M: www.a4m.com

BioTE: www.BioTEmedical.com

Iowa Bioidentical Specialists: www.Iowabioidentical.com

EndocrineWeb: www.endocrineweb.com

Hakala Research: www.hakalalabs.com (iodine testing)

Urine hormone testing is also available through:

Genova Diagnostics: www.gdx.net

Precision Analytical: https://dutchtest.com/resource/testing-matrix/

Meridian Valley Lab: meridianvalleylab.com

Chapter 6 References

1. Brownstein, David. *Overcoming Thyroid Disorders*. ed. 2. West Bloomfield, Michigan: Medical Alternatives Press, 2002.

2. Brownstein, David. *Salt your way to health*. West Bloomfield, Michigan: Medical Alternatives Press (2010).

3. Brownstein, David. *Iodine, Why You Need It. Why You Can't Live Without It*. West Bloomfield, Michigan: Medical Alternatives Press (2014).

4. Bunevicius, R., G. Kazanavicius, R. Zalinkevicius, and A.J. Prange Jr. "Effects of thyroxine as compared with thyroxine plus triiodothyronine in patients with hypothyroidism." *New England Journal of Medicine* 6. no. 340 (1999): 424–9.

5. Collins, Joseph. *Discover Your Menopause Type*. Three Rivers Press, 2002.

6. Donovitz, Gary. *Age Healthier Live Happier*. Orlando, Florida: Celebrity Press, 2015.

7. Gaitonde, David Y., Kevin D. Rowley, and Lori B. Sweeney. "Hypothyroidism: An Update." *American Family Physician* 3. no. 86 (2012): 244-251. http://www.aafp.org/afp/2012/0801/p244.html.

8. Gärtner, Roland, B.C. Gasnier, J.W. Dietrich, B. Krebs, M.W. Angstwurm. "Selenium supplementation in patients with autoimmune thyroiditis decreases thyroid peroxidase antibodies concentrations." *The Journal of Clinical Endocrinology and Metabolism* 4. no. 87 (2002): 1687–91.

9. Jefferies, William. *Safe Use of Cortisol, 3rd Edition.* Springfield, Illinois: Charles C Thomas, 2004.

10. Hertoghe, Thierry. *The Hormone Handbook.* Windhof, Luxembourg: International Medical Books, 2010.

11. Kelly, Tamas, Lawrence Denmark, and Daniel Lieberman. "Elevated levels of circulating thyroid hormone do not cause the medical sequelae of hyperthyroidism." *Progress in Neuro-Psychopharmacology and Biological Psychiatry*. vol. 71 (2016): 1–6.

12. Khera, M., D. Crawford, A. Morales, A. Salonia, and A. Morgentaler. "A new era of testosterone and prostate cancer: From physiology to clinical implications," *European Urology* 65. (2013): 114–123.

13. Kharrazian, Datis. *Why Do I Still Have Thyroid Symptoms? When My Labs Are Normal.* Garden City, New York: Morgan James Publishing (2010).

14. Lord, Richard, and Cheryl Burdette. *Measuring Urinary Estrogen Metabolites for Cancer Risk Assessment.* Metametrix Clinical Laboratory Department of Science and Education, 2006. http://www.metametrix.com/files/learning-center/articles/Estrogen-Metabolites.pdf.

15. Farrow, Lynne. *The Iodine Crisis: What You Don't Know About Iodine Can Wreck Your Life.* Devon Press, 2013.

16. Mayo Clinic. "Menopause." mayoclinc.org (2017). https://www.mayoclinic.org/diseases-conditions/menopause/symptoms-causes/syc-20353397.

17. Mishell, Daniel. "A Clinical Study of Estrogenic Therapy with Pellet Implantation." *American Journal of Obstetrics and Gynecology* 6, no. 41 (1941): 1009-1017. http://www.ajog.org/article/S0002-9378(16)40840-9/fulltext.

18. Morgentaler, Abraham, et al. "Fundamental concepts regarding testosterone deficiency and treatment: International expert consensus resolutions." *Mayo Clinic Proceedings* 7, no. 91. (2016): 881–896.

19. Morgentaler, A., and A. Traish. "Shifting the paradigm of testosterone and prostate cancer: The saturation model and the limits of androgen-dependent growth." *European Urology* 55. (2009): 310–321.

20. Moskowitz, Deborah. "A comprehensive review of the safety and efficacy of bioidentical hormones for the management of menopause and related health risks." *Alternative Medicine Review* 3, no. 11. (2006): 208–222.

21. Singh, M., P. Francis, and M. Michael. (2011). "Tamoxifen, cytochrome p450 genes and breast cancer clinical outcomes." The Breast 20. (2011): 111-118.

22. Smith, Pam. *What You Must Know About Vitamins, Minerals, Herbs, and More: Choosing the Nutrients That Are Right for You*. Garden City Park, New York: Square One Publishers, 2008.

23. Wehrwein, Peter. "Astounding increase in antidepressant use by Americans." *Harvard Health Publishing* (2011). https://www.health.harvard.edu/blog/astounding-increase-in-antidepressant-use-by-americans-201110203624.

24. Wentz, Izabella. *Hashimoto's Thyroiditis: Lifestyle Interventions for Finding and Treating the Root Cause*. Wentz, LLC, 2013.

25. Zeligs, M.A., P.K. Brownstone, M.E. Sharp, K. Westerlind, S. Wilson, and S. Johns. "Managing cyclical mastalgia with absorbable diindolylmethane: A randomized placebo-controlled trial." *Journal of the American Nutraceutical Association* 1, no. 8 (2011): 10–20.

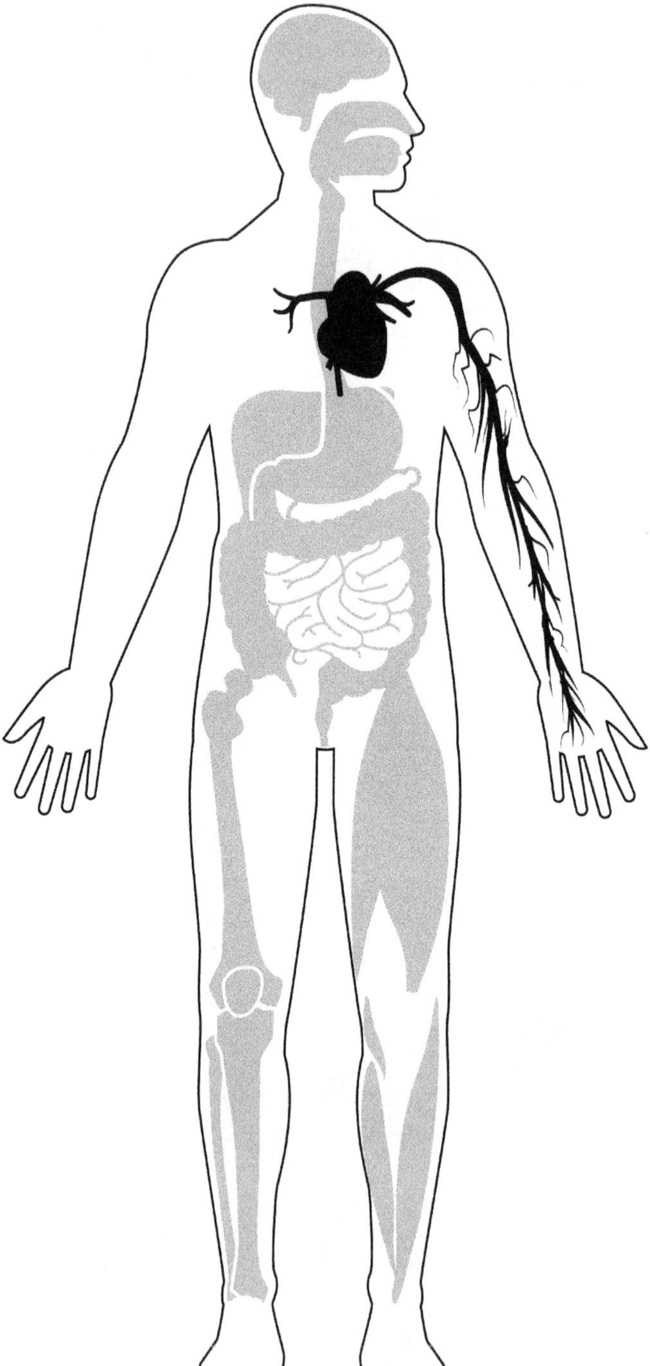

CHAPTER 7

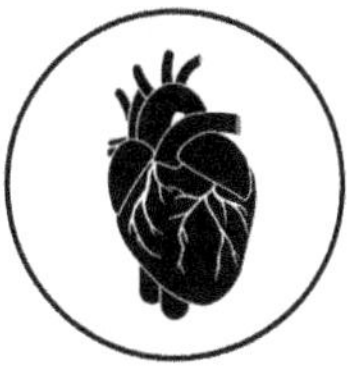

CLOG-FREE PLUMBING: REDUCING CARDIOVASCULAR DISEASE

Inflammation—a fast track to heart disease.

—Mark Houston, MD, MS

Have you ever worried during a heavy rain if your sump pump is going to hold up? Do you spend enormous amounts of time winterizing your home so your pipes don't freeze or burst, leaving you with water damage? If you've experienced water damage, you know how dreadful and expensive it can be.

The water pressure in a home is also important. Multiple factors affect water pressure, including the size and length of the pipework along with factors such as calcium buildup inside your pipes. It's the same with your arteries: you want your arteries clear, and you want your heart (your body's sump pump) to keep things running smoothly.

You depend on water for everyday activities—bathing, brushing teeth, washing hands, cleaning the dishes, doing laundry—so you need your plumbing to get you through the day clog-free. Most individuals also understand that grease poured down the drain will inevitably harden, leading to a clog. Similarly, our bodies depend on blood, which carries oxygen and vital nutrients to all our organs. And just like clogged pipes in a house can lead to problems, clogged veins can lead to serious health consequences.

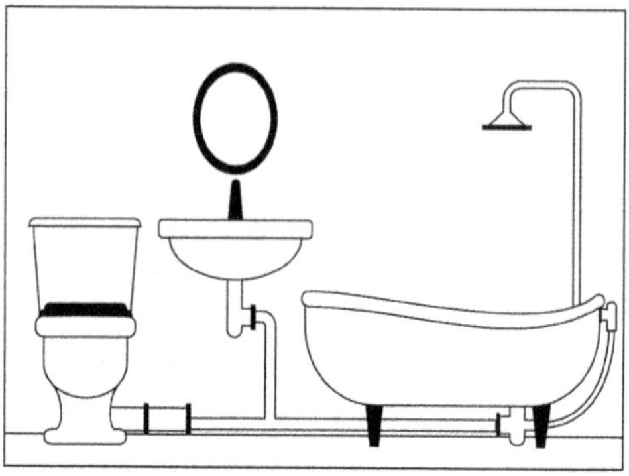

Unfortunately, the cardiovascular system is one system that does not always alert you with symptoms until you are in the danger zone. By the time you experience chest pains, you likely have had plaque building up in your arteries for some time. There aren't always symptoms for high blood pressure or high cholesterol, either. Cardiovascular disease (CVD) has been known as the silent killer.

Clogged arteries are a result of cholesterol, fat, calcium, white blood cells, and platelets combining, forming a glue-like plaque. This plaque then slowly builds up on the endothelium, the lining of your blood vessels. It can harden the arteries, causing them to narrow. When there is a narrowing of the arteries, blood can't flow through the space as easily and your blood pressure rises. This buildup of plaque is often referred to as atherosclerosis, which can lead to heart disease, heart attack, and stroke, all forms of coronary heart disease (CHD). Chronic inflammation and oxidation (like how an apple slice turns brown) drives the process forward. Within this chapter I will be discussing how to reduce risk not only for CHD, but for all CVD. Keeping CVD under control requires reducing the plaque, reducing inflammation, and reducing oxidation. In fact, integrative cardiologist Mark Houston states that any treatment of cardiovascular disease that doesn't acknowledge inflammation and its role is obsolete (Houston 2012).

A patient of mine, Sarah, came from a family with a strong history of cardiovascular disease. She came to see me when she was in her thirties, after all of her older brothers and her father had already passed away from heart attacks. Interestingly, none of them had high cholesterol, including Sarah. But she had been placed on a statin medication because she was told it would reduce her risk. She didn't tolerate it at all. It made her tired and achy. She came to our clinic with the high fear that she, too, would die an early death. She was exercising four to five days a week, and eating what she thought was a clean diet. She had read that individuals with both high and low cholesterol die of heart attacks. She knew there had to be more to her story.

CARDIOVASCULAR SYSTEM

The cardiovascular system is part of the larger circulatory system, hence its name, which refers to its role of "circulating" fluids throughout the body. The circulatory system includes the cardiovascular and lymphatic systems. The cardiovascular system circulates blood throughout the body, and the lymphatic system moves the lymph, which is a clear fluid that's similar to plasma in blood. I discussed the lymphatics important role in chapter 5.

Blood carries nutrients from the foods you eat and oxygen from the air you breathe to your cells. The blood then transports waste products from those cells to be removed from the body. Blood also contains hormones and various cells that help to fight infections. Because of these activities, our blood has been called the "river of life."

CARDIOVASCULAR SYSTEM

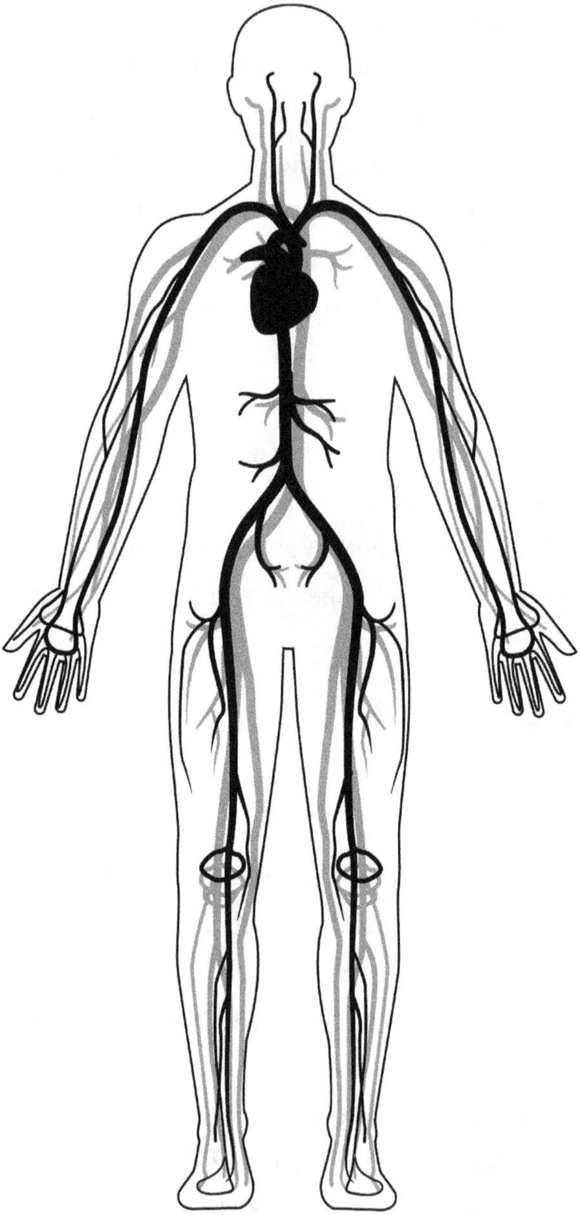

The cardiovascular system includes the heart (the organ that pumps the blood) and blood vessels. The arteries carry blood away from the heart. The veins return blood to the heart. Capillaries lie between the arteries and veins, connecting them. When healthy, your arteries are flexible. As heart disease sets in, they become more hardened, less flexible.

HEART DISEASE

It's no secret that diseases of the cardiovascular system are the leading cause of death in both men and women in the United States. According to the CDC, **one in every four deaths** is from cardiovascular disease. Specifically, CVD is the most common type of CVD. Every year, three quarters of a million Americans experience a heart attack. Annually, approximately one in every six US health care dollars is spent on cardiovascular disease. In 2011, heart disease and stroke cost the nation an estimated $316.6 billion in health care costs and lost productivity (CDC 2017).

What is heart disease? Heart disease occurs when there is damage to the lining and inner layers of the vascular system. According to the National Institute for Health, the top contributors to this lining damage include smoking, high cholesterol, high blood pressure, a high sugar diet leading to insulin resistance, and blood vessel inflammation. Where this damage is present, plaque begins to build up. The danger occurs when the plaque hardens and narrows the arteries, which reduces the flow of oxygen-rich blood to the heart. That can then manifest as chest pain. Also, if the plaque breaks open, platelets start clumping or sticking to the site of the injury, which can form a blood clot, further narrowing the artery. If the location of the clot is in the lung, it causes a pulmonary embolism. If that clot occurs in the heart, it causes a heart attack. If it occludes blood flow to the brain, it can cause a stroke.

RISK FACTORS FOR CARDIOVASCULAR DISEASE

Again, the top contributors to cardiovascular disease are smoking, high blood pressure, insulin resistance and diabetes, high cholesterol, and overall blood vessel inflammation. Sarah needed to be assessed for all of the above, not just for cholesterol (SpectraCell 2017). According to the National Cholesterol Education Program guidelines, Sarah is typical to many Americans. Fifty percent of the people that present to the emergency room with confirmed strokes or heart attacks have had normal blood pressure and cholesterol (SpectraCell 2017).

Smoking damages every organ in your body. Not only is it toxic for your body, containing many hazardous chemicals, it also damages the heart and narrows the vessels. It also increases blood pressure and reduces good cholesterol.

Blood pressure is the pressure of blood flow in your body. The optimal blood pressure measurement is < 120 over < 80 mmHg. If your reading is higher, you could be at increased risk for CVD. The medical term for high blood pressure is **hypertension**. It is often called the silent killer, because there are frequently no major symptoms until blood pressure is in a very dangerous range. It can cause nosebleeds, headaches, or dizziness. High blood pressure occurs in part due to **endothelial dysfunction**, which is a fancy term for inflammation of the inner lining of blood vessels.

In adults, a body mass index (BMI) of 18.5 to 24.9 is considered normal. A BMI greater than twenty-five is overweight, and greater than thirty is considered obese. The prevalence of obesity in the

United States has been increasing and continues to rise. In 2015, only seven states had a population with normal BMIs (BRFSS 2015). All the rest were considered overweight, obese, or extremely obese (BRFSS 2015).

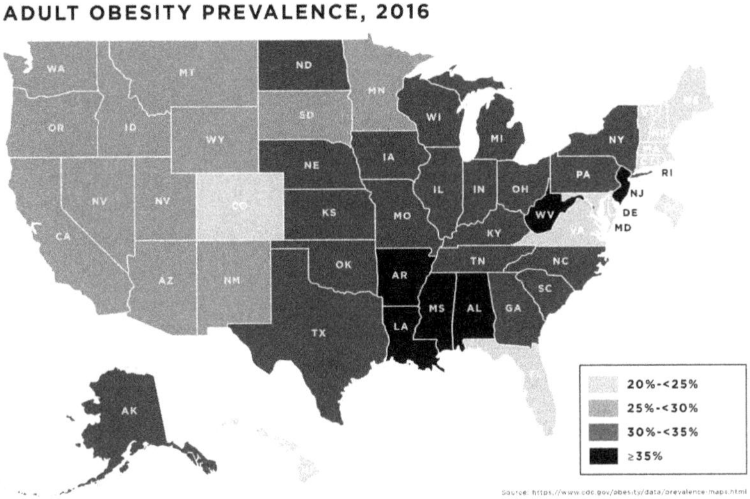

Prevalence of Self-Reported Obesity Among U.S. Adults by State and Territory (BRFSS 2015)

Obesity increases risk for heart disease, in part because it increases risk for insulin resistance and ultimately diabetes. However, you don't have to be obese to have insulin resistance. In fact, more than one fourth of individuals studied were insulin resistant with a normal BMI (Wildman 2008). **Insulin** is a hormone produced by the beta cells of the pancreas, and helps with the metabolism of carbohydrates, fats, and proteins. It is essential for the body's utilization of glucose for energy. Insulin resistance (IR) happens when the body's cells become resistant to the effects of insulin. When this happens, the pancreas produces more and more insulin, until it can no longer produce sufficient insulin for the body's demands, and then blood glucose (sugar) levels increase. Insulin resistance is known as "**pre-diabetes.**" Often there are no major signs of insulin resistance until the individual develops **type two diabetes**. These symptoms include excessive thirst, frequent urination, weight gain, fatigue, foul smelling urine, and a darkening of skin under the chin, in the groin, or in the armpits. In the United States, twenty-nine million people (9.3 percent) have diabetes. The total estimated cost of diagnosed diabetes in 2012 was $245 billion, including $176 billion in direct medical costs, and $69 billion in reduced productivity (ADA 2017).

Metabolic syndrome

Having a combination of risk factors can place an individual at risk for metabolic syndrome, which is also a risk for CVD. In order to meet criteria for metabolic syndrome, you must have at least three out of five of the following factors:

- excess fat in the stomach area (central obesity)
- high blood pressure
- high triglyceride levels
- low HDL (helpful or good) cholesterol level
- high fasting blood sugar (early sign of diabetes)

It's fairly easy to determine if you have central obesity. First, measure your waist circumference. For men to be considered low risk, their waist should be less than 37 inches, and for women, below 31.5 inches. If a man's waist is 37.1 to 39.9 inches, or a woman's is 31.6 to 34.9 inches, they are considered at intermediate risk. **High risk** is over 40 inches for a man, and above 35 inches for a woman.

The causes of high blood pressure specifically are similar to those of heart disease, including smoking, lack of physical exercise, high alcohol intake, poor nutrition with a diet high in processed foods, genetics, sleep apnea, adrenal and thyroid disorders, and stress.

TESTING FOR CARDIOMETABOLIC SYNDROME

Cardiometabolic syndrome (CMS) is a combination of interrelated risk factors that promote the development of atherosclerosis (fatty deposits on artery walls) and type two diabetes mellitus. Your cardiometabolic risk refers to your chances of having heart disease, strokes, or diabetes.

There are several labs that now offer advanced testing to further assess cardiometabolic risk. These labs offer advanced lipid assessments, often called a lipoprotein particle analysis, as well as comprehensive insulin/diabetes testing. These labs can produce subfraction measurements of cholesterol rather than the basic lipid panel you may be familiar with. Think of **lipoproteins** as transporters or carriers of cholesterol and triglycerides through the bloodstream. The *number* and *size* of these lipoproteins may better predict their **atherogenic potential**—or, their potential to promote the formation of fatty plaques in the arties. The main lab I use for this testing is True Health Diagnostics. I have also used SpectraCell Laboratories.

Cholesterol

Before we break down the lipid panel, let me first explain total cholesterol. This is the total amount of cholesterol circulating in your blood. It includes both the good and bad cholesterol, as well as triglycerides. Typically the goal is to have cholesterol <200 mg/dL. You need a decent amount of cholesterol to help cell membranes and to make hormones. When I need to assess if a patient with low testosterone has the necessary building blocks for hormone production or not, one of the first tests I run is a cholesterol panel, especially if they are on cholesterol lowering medications (statins).

Next, let's discuss the "good guys"—the helpers. **High density lipoproteins (HDLs)** are known as the good cholesterol. They help remove damaged lipids, bringing them back to the liver for excretion. Low HDL is a risk factor if below 40 mg/dL in men and 50 mg/dL in women.

Next, we have **low density lipoproteins (LDL)**. Think of them as "lousy" or bad cholesterol. A basic goal is to keep them <100 mg/dL. Many doctors treat patients based on the LDL number. This number doesn't always translate into the patient's risk. Two individuals with the same LDL number could have varying degrees of risk, because their particles and inflammation could be different. Statin medications reduce **total LDL cholesterol (LDL-C)**, but not necessarily particles. Large clinical trials have proven **LDL particles (LDL-P)** are more predictive of cardiovascular disease. The risk is more related to the total amount of bad (P) particle markers. The American Diabetes Association and the American College of Cardiology endorse LDL-P as the biggest risk-inducing marker. A general goal for particle number is less than a thousand. The lower the particle number, the less likely you are to build plaque in your arteries.

We can now also take testing a step further and assess **small dense LDL-C (sdLDL-C)**. This measures the very small, dense particles, which are also very risk inducing, as the small particles are the ones that often stick to the vessel wall and develop into a fatty streak, starting the plaque-building process. These can break off and lead to a clot. You want to have larger particles, not smaller ones. Keep your sdLDL <20 mg/dL.

Additionally, you can have your particle pattern determined. Pattern A has more *large* LDL particles, which are less risk-inducing compared to pattern B, having *small* LDL particles, which are more risk inducing.

	GOAL
BODY MASS INDEX	18.5-24.9
TOTAL CHOLESTEROL	<200 mg/dL
HDL FEMALE	>40 mg/dL
HDL MALE	>50 mg/dL
LDL	<100 mg/dL
sdLDL	<20 mg/dL
TRIDLYGERIDES	<150 mg/dL
FIBRINOGEN	<350 mg/dL
HS-CRP	<1 mg/dL
HOMOCYSTEINE	<10 umol/L
Lp-PLA2	<200 ng/mL
Lp (a)	<30 mg/dL
MPO	<400 pmol/L
SED RATE	<20 mm/hour
INSULIN	<10 Miu/L
OMEGA 3:6 RATIO	>8% (varies)

KEY

mg/dL	milligrams per deciliter
umol/L	micromoles per liter
ng/mL	nanograms per milliliter
pmol/L	picomoles per liter
mIU/L	milli-international units per liter

Triglycerides

Triglycerides are simply fats in the blood. "Tri" means three, so triglycerides are three glyerol molecules together, which makes what we often call fats. Excess calories, alcohol, or sugar in the body turns into triglycerides, which can stick to vessel walls as well, promoting plaque, getting larger and thicker, and eventually breaking off and causing a clot. Typically, the higher the triglycerides, the lower the good HDL cholesterol. Also, as triglycerides rise, the lousy LDL particles tend to get smaller, thus more risk inducing. Your goal is to keep triglycerides <150 mg/dL. If elevated, they are an additional independent risk factor for cardiovascular disease.

INFLAMMATORY MARKERS

If you've only had your cholesterol panel checked, but never had any inflammatory markers assessed, your provider could be missing an important assessment of your CVD risk. A comprehensive cardiovascular assessment should also include the following inflammatory markers. Because this can be a silent disease, these markers are your "signs" of inflammation.

Fibrinogen

Fibrinogen is a sticky substance that promotes blood clotting. It's an important part of our body's repair system. However, if your fibrinogen is high, it can be an indication that damage has occurred. The thicker the blood, the more stress on the heart to circulate it. Your goal should be <350 mg/dL.

Highly Sensitive C-Reactive Protein (hs-CRP)

CRP rises in the body when inflammation is occurring. That can occur due to any infection, such as a common cold. Hs-CRP shows inflammation specific to the heart and is used to predict the risk of developing CVD. The higher the inflammation, the greater the chance for plaque rupturing, forming a clot. The pieces that break away can also migrate to smaller arteries, where they can block blood flow completely. This process can cause those tissues that are supplied by that artery to die. When that happens in the coronary arteries, it causes a heart attack. When it happens in the arteries of the brain, it causes a stroke. Your goal is less than 1 mg/L.

Homocysteine

Homocysteine is a sulfur-bearing amino acid that can increase risk for CVD, since high levels can increase plaque formation. There are no symptoms of high homocysteine levels; however, high levels have been associated with B vitamin deficiency status, kidney and liver disease, thyroid conditions, Alzheimer's disease, depression, erectile dysfunction, and some ocular diseases. If my patients have high homocysteine levels, I then typically test them to see if they have an MTHFR variant (as discussed in chapter 3), and then I trial them on B6, B9, and B12 supplements to help reduce this level. Keep your level <10.8 mol/L.

Lipoprotein Associated Phospholipase A2 (Lp-PLA 2)

Associated with bad cholesterol, Lp-PLA 2 is an enzymatic specific marker of inflammation in the coronary arteries. It is a marker for oxidation, and it accumulates in plaque, thus indicating that plaque is actively building up. Your goal is <200 ng/mL. Levels over 200 are highly correlated with **endothelial dysfunction,** which increases risk for CVD.

Lipoprotein(a)

Lipoprotein(a) or Lp(a) is the worst lipoprotein marker. It is an inherited or genetic trait that independently increases your risk for heart disease. It's been called the "deadly" cholesterol because it is plaque promoting and plaque forming. Unfortunately, this marker doesn't respond to diet or lifestyle changes. Niacin is one of the only available interventions that can help reduce it. Raising estradiol levels in postmenopausal women can also help. Your goal should be <30 mg/dL.

Myeloperoxidase (MPO)

MPO is an enzyme made by white blood cells when the body has an injury or infection. It produces a type of "bleach" that damages the arteries leading to unstable plaque. However, it oxidizes LDL, which also increases risk for plaque. Your goal should be <400 pmol/L.

Omega-3 Index

There are several companies on the market that can now measure an omega-3 index. This is an index of the omega 3 fatty acids (EPA/DHA) in your red blood cells. This index is included in the nutritional evaluation mentioned in chapter 4. It is also included in a comprehensive particle analysis through True Health Diagnostics. In chapters 1 and 4, I discuss the importance of omegas for healing the gut and reducing inflammation. Omegas are also excellent for reducing cardiovascular inflammation. Your goal is to have higher omega-3s in your blood compared to omega-6s.

The risk of heart disease rises when there's an increase in omega-6s in our diets. Farmers feed their cows soybeans and corn (omega-6s), and these omega-6s also end up being a major component of vegetable oils. Hydrogenation turns vegetable oils into solids, improves flavor, and supposedly increases its uses for cooking. Many restaurants use hydrogenated oils, as their shelf life is longer. When oils are hydrogenated, omega-3s are destroyed. Hydrogenated oils are the worst fats you can consume, worse than the bad saturated fats. Hydrogenation doesn't exist in nature. Our bodies can't easily digest these oils. Billions of dollars have been spent creating drugs to suppress omega-6 inflammatory signaling. What if a simple change in diet to reduce omega-6s and increase omega-3s could eliminate the need for drugs? A fish oil supplement loaded with omega-3s can help.

In her book *Queen of Fats,* Susan Allport makes a case for why cardiovascular disease is on the rise: because fats have been removed from our diets. She discusses in-depth the study of the Inuit Eskimos' diet, concluding that the diet reduced the risk of heart disease (Allport 2006). Nielson, Bang, and Dyerberg studied this population, and found that the time it took their blood to clot was much longer than other populations (ibid). Their research found that these Inuit Eskimos had higher amounts of EPA in their blood from the seal blubber they had been eating (ibid).

How do omega-3s reduce inflammation? They block the production of prostaglandins. They inhibit the same COX and LOX enzymes that drugs like ibuprofen do. They reduce platelet aggregation, meaning they inhibit platelets from sticking together and forming a clot.

Having an optimal omega-3 index is essential for reducing inflammation, blood pressure, glucose, clotting, and triglycerides. Omega-3 fatty acids have been shown in epidemiological and clinical trials to reduce the incidence of CVD. Literally, the higher your omega-3 index, the lower your risk for mortality and morbidity—not only for CVD, but for other conditions as well.

Sedimentation Rate (sed rate)

An erythrocyte sedimentation rate (sed rate) reveals inflammation in your body. It can help diagnose various inflammatory conditions, but it is usually combined with other tests, like the ones mentioned above. Your goal is to keep your sed rate <20 mm/hr.

Insulin

As mentioned earlier, high glucose can indicate insulin resistance. However, this can take years for glucose to flag a high or positive on your annual blood work. Having your provider check fasting insulin can help you more quickly identify insulin resistance. Insulin rises before glucose will. A perfect fasting insulin is 6 mIU/L.

Proinsulin

Proinsulin is the precursor to insulin. High levels have been seen in patients with insulin resistance, pancreatic tumors, and liver failure.

Nitric Oxide (NO)

Nitric oxide (NO) is a signaling molecule, a combination of nitrogen and oxygen. According to cardiologist Stephen Sinatra, NO promotes healthy dilation, or the opening of the veins and arteries so that blood can move through effectively. It can also help prevent red blood cells from sticking together, creating dangerous clots and blockages. "Your body naturally generates NO in the endothelium that lines the blood vessel walls. But in the early stages of arterial disease, this lining is damaged—which chokes off the production of NO, making the vessels vulnerable to inflammation and other negative factors" (drsinatra.com 2017). I highly recommend his books, including *The Sinatra Solution: Metabolic Cardiology* (2005), and *The Great Cholesterol Myth* (2012).

Impotence medications like Viagra act on the nitric oxide pathway. You may have heard of the medication nitroglycerin in the nitrate family, which is used to open blood vessels, increasing blood flow to the heart to reduce chest pains. Several medical journals, including the *New England Journal of Medicine*, have well established that high NO levels help increase blood flow, energy, and endurance. At my practice, we also offer a quick and easy saliva test, which measures the body's bioavailability of nitric oxide. High levels can indicate endurance and elevated performance, while low levels are associated with fatigue. I often see low NO levels in my patients with high blood pressure and erectile dysfunction. Ideally, prior to ever needing Viagra or nitroglycerine, it should be explored whether you have low NO levels so that they can be repleted. To learn more about NO, read Bryan and Zand's (2010) book, *The Nitric Oxide (NO) Solution*. Also of note, Viagra and nitrates should not be taken together.

To truly determine your cardiovascular risk, all the above levels should be assessed together. I look at the combination of risk factors with my patients to establish how aggressive we need to be to keep their pipes from clogging, also known as keeping their arteries clear!

HOW TO REDUCE YOUR CVD RISK

Currently, there are several strategies to help reduce risk for CVD. These include various pharmaceutical drugs, diets, exercise, and a number of nutraceutical products.

Drugs

There are several pharmaceutical options available to help lower cholesterol. Most individuals are familiar with the frequently prescribed statin medications for lowering cholesterol. These drugs alone are a $20 to $40 billion industry. These are HMG-CoA reductase inhibitors. They work by inhibiting the rate at which cholesterol is manufactured in the liver, and they can significantly reduce cholesterol. Reducing cholesterol, however, doesn't mean they reduce an individual's risk. It's been proposed that they may actually *only* reduce risk because they reduce inflammation. Additionally, side effects of these drugs range from mild muscle aches to severe muscle and kidney damage. This muscle aching is described in medicine as "myopathy."

Many patients who come to me have already tried statins without success, and with poor tolerability. Genetic testing exists to explore whether statins are essentially a good fit for the patient. Twenty-five percent of individuals have one copy of the **SLC01B1** genetic variant, which means they have increased risk for the side effects of statins coupled with the medication for lowering their cholesterol being less effective. Five percent of individuals have two copies of this mutation and have a greater risk for side effects and efficacy. For patients who already complain of muscle aches or who are concerned with the side effects, I often consider genetic testing to see if statins are a good fit.

A separate class of cholesterol absorption inhibitors exists, and these prevent or block the uptake of cholesterol from the small intestine into the blood. When cholesterol is blocked into the bloodstream, it stays in the lumen of the gut until it is excreted, essentially pooped out. The most commonly prescribed drug in this class I have used is Zetia (ezetimibe). Additionally, plant sterols can be used to help as well.

A second strength in having a thorough particle analysis run through True Health Diagnostics is that it actually tests for sterols, which helps the clinician decide the best fit for the patient. If sterol *absorption* markers are high, then a drug like Zetia is a better fit for the patient. If sterol *synthesis* markers are high, red yeast rice or statin medication would be a better fit. For instance, does the cholesterol manufacturing need to be blocked in the liver, or does it need to be blocked in the gut from entering the bloodstream? A regular lipid panel most certainly doesn't answer that question. The advanced testing helps identify what supplements and/or drugs are the best fit for the patient tested.

Lastly, if you have to take drugs, remember to take the nutrients they deplete from your body.

Diet

Countless books have been written on various diets to help reduce cardiovascular diseases. We know increased weight is directly linked to a slew of health conditions, so what is the best diet for weight loss?

The Mediterranean diet is one of the world's healthiest diets. This diet is abundant in fruits, vegetables, whole grains, legumes, and olive oil. It is low in red meat (which contains more saturated fat) and instead features fish and poultry—lean sources of protein. Red wine can be consumed regularly, but in modest amounts.

I tend to agree that this diet can help reduce CVD risk, and can help with weight loss and diabetes. However, we are all genetically different, and a diet that is best for one individual may not be the best for another. Since inflammation places you at high risk, avoiding foods that are inflammatory for you (based on the testing mentioned in chapter 1) will help keep your inflammatory markers down. For instance, whole grains may be beneficial for you, but not the glutinous grains if you have a gluten sensitivity.

William Davis, the cardiologist who wrote the book *Wheat Belly*, took his patients off all grains and found that many lost weight, reduced their appetites, improved insulin resistance, and resolved diabetes. Additionally, they lowered their cholesterol and reduced their risk of heart disease.

As I mentioned earlier in the book, you need to think about what your food eats. Does it consume grain high in omega-6s, or is it pasture raised, consuming greens, like grass, high in omega-3s? This includes your eggs. It's been said that our eggs contain a tenth of the omegas in eggs in other countries. Why? Our chickens are fed grains like corn, not grass.

Increase omega-3s in your diet through sources such as enriched organic eggs from organic free-range, grass-fed, pasture-raised chickens. Eat wild-caught fish every week. Avoid omega-6s like safflower, sunflower, corn, canola, walnut, and soybean oils. If you consume them, verify they are not hydrogenated. Choose to consume free-range, grass-fed chicken, beef, bison, and pork.

Overall, work to reduce bad saturated fats like hydrogenated oils, and instead opt for nonhydrogenated oils and unsaturated fats. You must read labels to avoid these. Specifically, avoid margarine, frostings, shortenings, donuts, whipped toppings, and creamers that contain these.

Many trials have shown that garlic has cardiovascular benefits. Celery is also a natural diuretic, which can help reduce blood pressure. Consuming pomegranate juice daily can help reduce blood pressure as well.

Increase fiber in your diet. In chapter 1, I mention how fiber can help with gut health, and in chapter 5 I mention that fiber can help bind to toxins to help you get rid of them. Fiber can also help bind cholesterol. Soluble fiber like guar gum, psyllium, and oat bran can help to reduce cholesterol and blood pressure. Consider adding gluten free oatmeal as a breakfast option.

Increase fruits and green veggies on a daily basis. Eat as many veggies as you possibly can. They are low in calories, rich in nutrients like vitamins, minerals, and antioxidants, and often contain fiber.

Salt is also not bad. Salt is necessary for every cell in your body to function. However, there is a difference between processed table salt loaded with chemicals and robbed of any trace minerals, which ultimately increases your blood pressure, and a pure sea salt loaded with trace minerals. Avoid the former. I prefer Himalayan or Celtic Keltic sea salt.

I actually have a family member who discovered that every time he stopped drinking alcohol his blood pressure normalized. Consume alcohol in moderation. Keep liquor consumption at less than two ounces per day, beer less than twenty-four ounces per day, and wine less than ten ounces per day. Remember that alcohol turns to sugar in your body, which raises triglycerides.

Reduce processed sugar and carbohydrates. The glycemic index (GI) is the ranking of carbohydrates according to the amount they will increase your blood glucose *after eating.* "Foods with a high GI are those which are rapidly digested and absorbed and result in marked fluctuations in blood sugar levels. Low-GI foods, by virtue of their slow digestion and absorption, produce gradual rises in blood sugar and insulin levels, and have proven benefits for health" (glycemicindex.com). Consider consuming low glycemic index foods to help stabilize your blood sugar levels. There are various smartphone apps and websites that allow you to search the GI of any food. In *Wheat Belly*, Davis discusses an "explosion of small LDL particles" with carbohydrate intake, concluding that one of the most important lifestyle interventions for reducing LDL particles—and thus CVD—is to get the carbs, specifically glutinous wheat, out of your diet entirely (Davis 2011, 156).

Exercise

Of course, exercise helps prevent CVD as well as diabetes. Specific recommendations constantly vary. Current recommendations for the general population are to participate in a minimum of thirty minutes of moderate physical activity at least five days weekly. If one is trying to lose weight, increase the workout to sixty minutes a day. Many of my patients tell me they walk their dog thirty to forty minutes a day but still aren't losing weight. They also aren't sweating, and aren't getting their heart rates up. I often have to explain to them that they are only covering the basics. To make progress, they need to do *more* than they have been doing. Comprehensive exercise should incorporate aerobic exercise with resistance or strength training. Exercise should also include flexibility (stretching) and balance movements. Exercise naturally increases NO levels and helps with blood flow.

> **WARNING:** If you have an existing heart condition or abnormal blood pressure, please consult your health care professional before taking supplements to increase nitric oxide levels.

NUTRACEUTICAL SUPPLEMENTS TO HELP REDUCE CVD

Various high-quality nutraceutical products can be very effective at reducing glucose, blood pressure, and cholesterol. All the discussed nutrients should be dosed by your provider based on your personal needs.

Coenzyme Q10 (CoQ10) is a potent antioxidant that can help to reduce blood pressure 15/10 mm Hg points, on average. Remember, CoQ10 is mentioned in chapter 4 as being important to replete when on cardiovascular drugs, and CoQ10 levels can be tested to help perfect dosing. We carry two LB CoQ10 products, a 100 mg and a 300 mg.

Berberine is a plant extract, a natural alkaloid, with several beneficial properties. Clinical trials have demonstrated that berberine can help reduce blood pressure, cholesterol, triglycerides and glucose, as well as maintain insulin and keep the heart in regular rhythm. Dosing is typically 500 mg twice daily. Berberine has also been shown to be as effective as one gram of metformin in clinical trials. In fact, it also reduced liver function better than metformin. Our LB product is Berberine Support.

Sardinia, Italy, is the second largest island in the Mediterranean, and one of the blue zones inhabiting many centenarians. Here the **citrus bergamot** fruit grows abundantly, and is a known staple of the Sardinian diet. Sardinians are said to drink one glass of bergamot juice daily, similar to Floridians drinking orange juice daily. Interestingly, Sardinians have a lower prevalence of cardiovascular disease and cholesterol. The bergamot's polyphenols help reduce oxidized LDL and reduce HMG-CoA reductase, while increasing HDL and particle size. In addition, bergamot doesn't deplete CoQ10 like statins do. Again, a typical dose would be one gram/day. When using bergamot products with my patients, I have noticed some source their product from the United States, but the best source for this product is Sardinia. This has produced the maximum results, and is the only source I use for my patients. Our LB product is Citrus Bergamot.

Carnitine, discussed in chapter 4, is excellent for the heart, because it transports fatty acids into cells for energy production.

The amino acid **L-arginine** is the precursor for the production of NO. It can also greatly help to reduce blood pressure. Many arginine products also contain L-citrulline, because it is recycled back into arginine, helping to make even more nitric oxide. Athletes use these to support the flow of blood and oxygen to the skeletal muscles, and to help remove exercise-induced lactic acid buildup, thus reducing fatigue and recovery time. Arginine doses can be increased from one gram up to five grams. Blood pressure should be monitored to verify it is not becoming too low. L-citrulline's popularity has been increasing, and it has been replacing arginine. It is one of the best options for sustained NO, also increasing endothelial function. I use this often in my patients with high blood pressure and erectile dysfunction. The LB product I use is NOX Support.

As Allport states, omega-3s should not just be thought of as an "important supplement that could PREVENT heart disease, but as a nutrient whose absence was helping to CAUSE heart disease" (Allport 2006, 83). The American Heart Association even recommends consumption of two servings of fish per week. Consume omega-3 supplements like our LB Omegas! Dosage can be determined based on your labs. For those with very high triglycerides, I often use doses as high at 4,000 mg EPA/DHA/day. Fish oil will also help reduce glucose and insulin, as well as raise your omega-3 index.

> **Omega-3s should not just be thought of as an "important supplement that could PREVENT heart disease, but as a nutrient whose absence was helping to CAUSE heart disease."**

The majority of Americans do not consume the recommended twenty-five to thirty-five grams of fiber per day. Examine your diet and count how many grams you are consuming per day. If you need to increase, don't start with that high of a dose. Start slow and work your way up.

D-Ribose is an extremely useful nutrient for cardiovascular health. It can be used to treat irregular heart rhythms, heart failure, and muscle pains from statin medications. It is excellent for athletes. It helps with recovery because it supplies the heart with the additional energy that it is often starving for. I typically dose it at five grams, one to three times per day.

Magnesium, discussed in previous chapters, is one of the first nutrients I place patients on with high blood pressure. That LB product I use is Magnesium Chelate.

Niacin (B3) can greatly help reduce triglycerides, sdLDL, and Lp(a), in addition to increasing HDL. Doses for these effects can range from 500 to 3,000 mg/day. Niacin can cause flushing, and can increase liver function tests, so the patient should be monitored through therapy. Inositol hexaniacinate (no-flush) niacin doesn't lower cholesterol, and for that reason shouldn't be used. There are some time-release niacin options available that are still effective, and also reduce the flushing effects. The preferred form is known as nicotinic acid. At my clinic, we carry an LB Time Release Niacin that has worked well for our patients.

As you age, so does your endothelium. With endothelial dysfunction, there is a deficiency in NO. With less NO, your endothelium can't repair, which increases risk for atherosclerosis. I often use a product called **Neo40** in my practice. It helps boost NO in order to help the arteries relax and expand while lowering blood pressure, keeping the arteries younger and more flexible. Neo40 helps stop formation of blood clots and helps lower cholesterol, and it can help reverse erectile dysfunction. I always test patients' levels first, and, depending on how low they are, start with one or work up to two lozenges daily. This should be done under supervision of a functional medicine provider. Don't take Neo40 if you have low blood pressure. This product contains the aforementioned citrulline.

Panthetine (B5) has also been shown to improve lipid profiles and reduce oxidation of LDL. Doses higher than mentioned in chapter 4 have been used to lower cholesterol. Doses as high as 900 mg/day have been used in clinical trials.

Plant sterols contain beta-sitosterols. They help to bind cholesterol in the gut. These are relatively safe to use. The dose is typically 1.3–2 g/day. We carry an LB plant sterols product.

Red Yeast Rice (RYR), also known as *Monascus purpureus* rice, is the fermented product on which rice is grown. It contains sterols, and can block HMG-CoA reductase, similar to statin medications. It is the natural botanical from which statin medications are derived. Depending on the manufacturer, the potency of the product can vary considerably. RYR can also raise liver function tests, so the patient should be monitored through therapy. Doses can range from 600 to 2,400 mg/day. Currently there is controversy over use of this product, since it also can contain mycotoxin citrinin. Many providers are shying away from using it, as there now exists options like bergamot.

Turmeric is mentioned in chapter 1 for reducing gut inflammation. It also can help reduce cardiovascular, vessel inflammation. Try incorporating this into your cooking habits. To reduce inflammation, you must consume >1,000 mg/day. Our LB product is Turmeric Support.

CONCLUSION

With Sarah, even if she "could" tolerate the statin medication, she still had additional risk factors that needed to be addressed. Through advanced cardiovascular assessment, we identified several elevated markers, which increased her risk for cardiovascular disease aside from her "normal cholesterol." She was found to have high homocysteine, and was homozygous for MTHFR C677T, one of the variants I discuss in chapter 3. She didn't smoke, didn't have high blood pressure, and wasn't insulin resistant, but her triglycerides were high, and her omega-3 index was low. She also had the most dangerous of risk factors—blood vessel inflammation. She had high CRP, and a high sedimentation (sed) rate.

Many of my patients, including myself, have thought their omega-3 index would be optimal because they took a fish oil supplement. I was surprised to find that I needed more than I was taking. I placed Sarah on 3,000 mg EPA/DHA/day, which reduced her triglycerides, raised her omega-3 index, and reduced her inflammation. She was also placed on LB MethylB Complex to help reduce her homocysteine. She was placed on LB Turmeric Support to help reduce that inflammation, and she started an exercise regimen. We retested her particle analysis in three months, and her homocysteine, CRP, sed rate, and triglycerides had all reduced, while her omega-3 index improved.

Hearing Sarah's story should raise a new awareness of other important markers that should be routinely assessed. This is an extremely important part of your Longevity Blueprint, because heart disease is the number one killer. Many patients think that if they eat clean, exercise, and balance their hormones they have done all they need to do for CV risk, and that's just not the case. Without testing, we don't know your true risk. Testing helps us identify what markers we need to improve on.

How can you keep your pipes clean? Get tested, assess your damage, see how close your pipes are to clogging. Ask your provider to order a comprehensive particle analysis. Treatment should be under a licensed provider, and should include nutrition, exercise, weight loss, smoking cessation, limiting alcohol and caffeine, using nutraceuticals, and, only if needed, drugs. You can reduce your cardiovascular risk by following your Longevity Blueprint.

Longevity Blueprint Nutraceutical Products

Here are my favorite LB nutrients:

- CoQ10 100
- CoQ10 300
- Omega-3s
- Berberine Support
- NOX Support
- Citrus Bergamot
- Magnesium Chelate
- Methyl B Complex
- Time Release Niacin
- Plant Sterols
- Turmeric Support

Chapter 7 Resources

Centers for Disease Control and Prevention: www.CDC.gov

Dr. Sinatra website: www.drsinatra.com

National Institutes of Health: www.nih.gov

Neo40 website: https://www.humann.com/

The University of Sydney glycemic index: www.glycemicindex.com

Laboratories

Spectracell: https://www.spectracell.com/

True Health Diagnostics: https://truehealthdiag.com/

Chapter 7 References

1. Allport, Susan. *The Queen of Fats.* London, England: University of California Press, 2006.
2. American Diabetes Association. "Cost of Diabetes." diabetes.org. Accessed April 22, 2017, http://www.diabetes.org/advocacy/news-events/cost-of-diabetes.html?referrer=https://www.google.com.
3. Bryan, Nathan, and Janet Zand. *The Nitric Oxide (NO) Solution.* Austin, Texas: Neogenesis, 2010.
4. Centers for Disease Control and Prevention. "Behavioral Risk Factor Surveillance System." cdc.gov. Accessed August 28, 2017, https://www.cdc.gov/brfss/index.html.
5. Centers for Disease Control and Prevention. "Heart Disease Facts." cdc.gov. August 2017, https://www.cdc.gov/heartdisease/facts.htm.
6. Davis, William. *Wheat Belly.* New York: Rodale, 2011.
7. University of Sydney Glycemic Index. "About Us." glycemicindex.com. May 2017, http://www.glycemicindex.com/about.php/.
8. Guilliams, Thomas. "Managing lipoprotein dyslipidemias through lifestyle and nutraceutical therapies." *The Standard* 1, no. 7. (2005): 1–11.

9. Houston, Mark. *What Your Doctor May Not Tell You About Heart Disease.* New York: Hachette Book Group, 2012.

10. Million Hearts. "Costs and Consequences." millionhearts.hhs.gov. Accessed April 21, 2017, https://millionhearts.hhs.gov/learn-prevent/cost-consequences.html.

11. Reddy, J. Kota. "Understanding your advanced cardiovascular profile report." Reddy Cardiac Wellness & Diabetes Reversal Center. Sugar Land: Texas, 2012

12. Sinatra, Stephen. "Nitric oxide benefits cardiovascular health." dr.sinatra.com. Accessed August 28, 2017, www.drsinatra.com/nitric-oxide-benefits-cardiovascular-health.

13. Sinatra, Stephen. *The Sinatra Solution: Metabolic Cardiology.* Laguna Beach, California: Basic Health Publications, 2011.

14. SpectraCell Laboratories. "Cardiovascular and Pre-Diabetes Test." spectracell.com (2017). https://www.spectracell.com/patients/patient-cardiometabolic-and-diabetes-testing/.

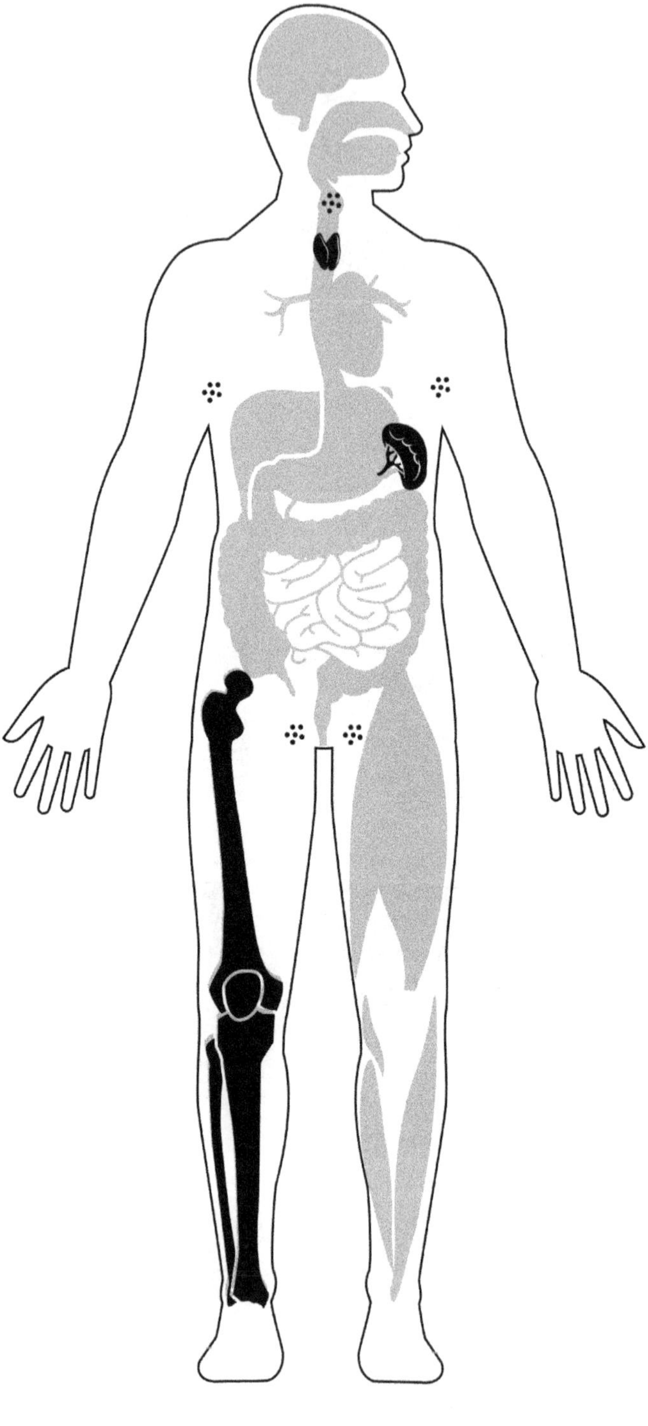

CHAPTER 8

MAINTAINING ROOF INTEGRITY: TREATING UNDERLYING INFECTIONS AND STRENGTHENING YOUR IMMUNE SYSTEM

"It's an important thing to realize that feeling powerless is detrimental to your health, and feeling like you can take some sort of action that could make a difference is crucial to your immune system."

—Kelly Turner, MD

I have experienced two major floods since living in Iowa. The worst was in 2008. At that time, my city, Cedar Rapids, was one of the hardest hit areas—if not the hardest hit. Our downtown was destroyed: businesses were lost, buildings had water up to the third floors, utilities were affected, and there were power outages. It took weeks for the water to recede. Although the short-term needs were evacuation, the long-term needs turned from rebuilding businesses and homes, to dealing with the health consequences of the water damaged buildings (WDBs).

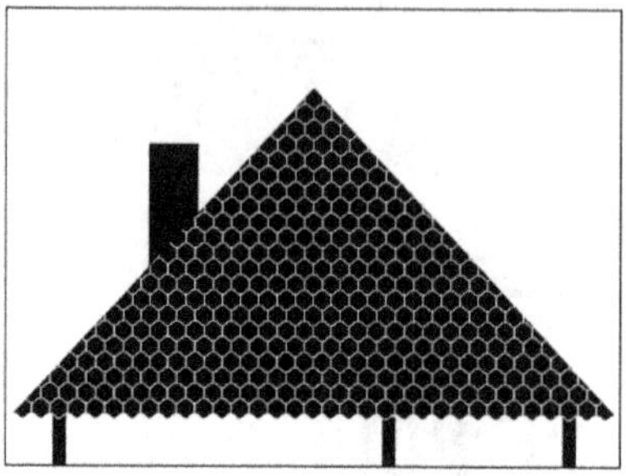

Although basements are particularly susceptible to flooding, water can also enter a home through a compromised roof. Without a solid roof, the home can easily be destroyed. If your roof leaks, your house can end up with water damage, which can lead to mold. This damage can impact the home's structural support, including the walls and floors. Think of the roof as a barrier to invaders in your home, just like your immune system acts as a barrier to infections in your body.

The same way water damage and mold can destroy your home, it can also destroy your health. I've had several patients since the flood of 2008 experience odd symptoms. Becky suffered from tinnitus and vertigo. She nearly always felt like she was spinning, and had terrible diarrhea several times a day. She was incredibly fatigued, and had terrible brain fog. Following what she had always done before for dizziness or headaches, she went to her chiropractor. However, this time, the adjustments were unsuccessful. She was suffering from chronic inflammatory response syndrome (CIRS) and didn't know it.

You may think you can skip over this chapter if you never get sick, don't have mold exposure, mono, or Lyme, but I encourage you to keep reading. You or someone you love may at some point experience a biotoxin illness, and believe me, if you do, you will be thankful you have read this chapter and have the needed resources to overcome it.

This next step in the Longevity Blueprint is the need to identify and treat current infections and to keep them at bay. Testing and treating for infections is one of the most difficult phases in this Longevity Blueprint, primarily because there aren't many providers truly specialized in being the detective, in being able to assess symptoms, order the appropriate and most progressive testing to diagnose, and then treat the patient correctly.

The most common infections I identify and treat in my clinic are the gastrointestinal infections: yeast, bacteria, and parasites. All three were discussed in greater detail in chapter 1.

In this chapter, I will briefly discuss the immune system as it relates to allergies, chronic inflammatory response syndrome (CIRS), lyme, mold, and viruses.

INTRODUCTION TO THE IMMUNE SYSTEM

The body's immune system is composed of a complex network of glands and cells that help detect invaders such as pathogens like viruses, bacteria, and parasites. Your body should also be able to identify what is "self" versus what is "non-self." The immune system is incredibly complex. Although I will not discuss cancer in this chapter, many of the immune boosters recommended can also help cancer patients.

The body's immune system is made of **bone marrow**—which produces immune cells—and organs like the thymus and spleen. Bone marrow is the flexible tissue in the inside of your bones that produces red blood cells through a process known as hematopoiesis. Bone marrow also produces lymphocytes.

The **thymus** is a triangular organ located in the middle of the thoracic cavity behind the sternum. The thymus trains your body's T cells (a type of white blood cell) to distinguish foreign antigens from those in your body.

Your **spleen** is fist shaped and located to the left of your stomach in the left part of your abdomen under your ribs. The spleen helps to filter blood as part of the immune system. It recycles old red blood cells and stores platelets and white blood cells, and it helps fight infections. An enlarged spleen is found in viral diseases like mono, liver disease, and blood cancers like lymphoma and leukemia.

Every day, invaders attempt to enter your body, and if they win and make it in, you get sick. Our primary defense is the **innate** immune response. It is composed of several **external barriers,** including mucous membranes, skin, and even stomach acid.

Your **skin** is your first line of defense. Your mucous membranes act as a permeable barrier to the interior of your body. Many infections invading the human body use this route. Think about it. What's the easiest way to get sick? Inhaling germs from another person, right? Skin is to your body what drywall is to your home. Both can tolerate a little damage, a few nicks and scrapes. But when your skin is deeply penetrated, or when a hole is made in the drywall, then what's underneath can begin to see damage.

Your lungs will cough and sneeze to literally eject pathogens and other irritants from your respiratory tract. Even tearing up and urinating helps to flush out pathogens. Mucus secreted by the respiratory and gastrointestinal tracts can help to trap and entangle invading microorganisms, too.

You also have white blood cells, known as leukocytes, and red blood cells. Think of white blood cells as soldiers ready to fight invaders. **White blood cells (WBCs)** are your second line of defense.

These are also involved in the innate immune response, whose job is to get the pathogens out. This response has no memory or lag time. Once an invader is in, the WBCs get to work. There are five types of WBCs: neutrophils, monocytes, lymphocytes, basophils, and eosinophils.

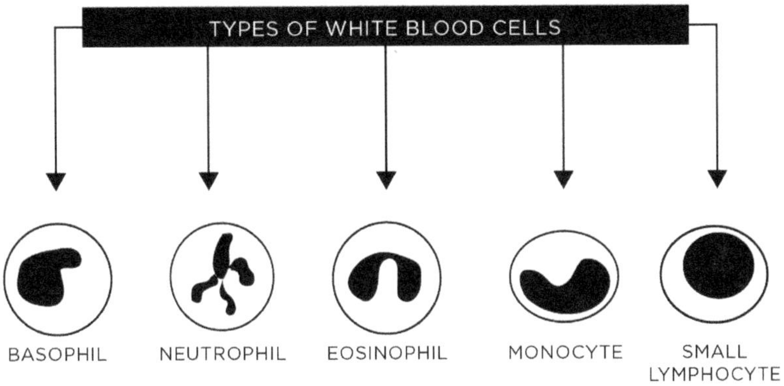

Neutrophils work to kill and digest bacteria and fungi. They are the most abundant type of WBCs, and the first responders to infection. Pus is an example of dead neutrophils.

Monocytes are the physically biggest WBCs. They help break down bacteria. They destroy what neutrophils don't. They can change or morph into cells called **macrophages,** which eat or gobble up remaining debris. They can literally engulf pathogens through a process called phagocytosis, or cell eating. Think of the macrophages as the housekeeper cleaning up the mess.

Lymphocytes create antibodies to defend against bacteria and viruses. There are two types of lymphocytes that provide immunity. **B lymphocyte cells** identify bacteria. They can then become a plasma cell that produces antibodies. Antibodies attach to the virus or pathogen to help trigger more WBCs to help destroy it. **T lymphocyte cells** destroy the invader. **Natural killer (NK) cells** are the most aggressive cells of our immune system, making up nearly 15 percent of the total circulating lymphocytes. They mature in the bone marrow, instead of in the thymus like other T cells. They are called natural killer cells because they do not need to recognize specific antibodies before releasing cytokines (strong intracellular signals), chemicals that program invaders to die. I like to think of them as the Navy SEALs of the immune system.

Basophils are small cells that sound the alarm to other cells when your body is infected. They can detect mold and make antibodies to destroy the foreign substance. They secrete chemicals such as histamine, and are responsible for hives, breathing difficulties, and asthma.

Eosinophils attack and kill bacteria and parasites, destroy cancer cells, and help with allergic responses as they trap and invade them.

On a complete blood count (CBC), which you've probably had tested several times in your life, high white blood cells suggest the presence of infection. You can assess all five types of WBCs on this lab. You can check lymphocytes as well. The CBC can help guide you if you have cancer, infections, allergies, or even parasites.

Remember in chapter 1 how I mention that the majority of our immune system is housed in our gut? There is overlap between the immune system and the gastrointestinal system, as the **gut-associated lymphoid tissue (GALT)** is a component of the mucosa-associated lymphoid tissue (MALT), which works within our immune system to protect our body from invasions within the gut. The GALT produces more plasma cells (which make antibodies) than the spleen, lymph nodes, and bone marrow combined.

Our **adaptive immune response** has a memory. This response takes time to adapt and to develop, but, once trained, these cells commit their training to memory. They can remember past exposure to pathogens. Adaptive immune system cells include leukocytes, called lymphocytes or B cells, which are involved in the **humoral immune response** through weapons known as antibodies, and T cells involved in **cell mediated immune response**. Both of these are derived from stem cells in bone marrow. Humoral immunity also involves complements, which are types of proteins that help destroy foreign invaders.

If both immune responses haven't eradicated the invaders, the liver tries to bind up the toxins in its bile ducts, and then it dumps the toxin-laden bile into the gallbladder. These toxins are then excreted into the small intestine. However, the toxins can be reabsorbed by a process called **enterohepatic circulation,** which means the toxins can get recirculated through the body and never truly get eliminated out of the bloodstream. These toxins can keep that innate immune system on overdrive, resulting in continued inflammation. More to come on this topic.

ALLERGIES

It's also nearly impossible to talk about our immune systems without mentioning allergies.

What are allergies? Some describe them as an overactive immune system. When we are exposed to an allergen, one of our immune cells—the mast cell—explodes and releases leukotrienes, inflammatory mediators, and histamine. This causes the vasodilation (opening) of vessels, as well as swelling, increasing flow of blood to that area. It also causes smooth muscle contraction, making breathing difficult, which can cause an asthma attack. It causes allergic symptoms like itchy eyes and runny noses, too. However, this is part of the natural response and healing process. Remember, steroids suppress the immune response, so they really suppress what is supposed to happen naturally. Antihistamines block histamine. There is a time and place for these drugs. However, ideally, it's better to calm the overactive immune system and prevent the allergenic cascade from occurring.

CHRONIC INFLAMMATORY RESPONSE SYNDROME

What becomes more difficult to treat are biotoxin-related illnesses. **Biotoxins** are poisonous substances produced by living organisms (bacteria, parasites, fungus) that can cross membranes. Even candida albicans (yeast) can generate gliotoxins, since they can be carried to the microglia in the brain. These all cause oxidative stress, and they can arrest cell cycles, essentially causing a slew of symptoms. According to Dr. Shoemaker, these biotoxins can cause an acute response or progress to chronic, systemic, inflammatory response syndrome (CIRS), acquired from exposure to the toxins (Shoemaker 2011). When I refer to mold exposure in this chapter, I'm simplifying the "interior environment of a water-damaged building with resident toxigenic organisms including, but not limited to, fungi, bacteria, actinomycetes, and mycobacteria" (Shoemaker 2011). Mold toxins account for 80 percent of these problems.

Interestingly, there is often overlap in symptoms of Lyme and mold patients. The NeuroQuant testing mentioned in chapter 2 can help to differentiate the true diagnosis.

You can become so inflamed from biotoxins that you can develop autoimmune diseases. Autoimmune diseases are a leading cause of death in middle-aged women. CIRS can manifest with a variety of symptoms in multiple body systems, including chronic fatigue, shortness of breath, weakness, mood swings, diarrhea, night sweats, poor temperature regulation, cramps, pains, stiffness, thirst, static shocks, problems focusing, light sensitivity, confusion, vertigo, tingling, numbness, ice pick pains, headaches, blurred vision, metallic taste, tremors, skin sensitivities, tearing, and coughing (Berndson et al. 2016).

The problem is that many pathogens can adapt to avoid detection, and many times an individual doesn't know their roof has been compromised and they've been "invaded" until years later.

CHRONIC INFLAMMATORY RESPONSE SYNDROME SYMPTOMS

- Fatigue
- Weakness
- Aches
- Muscle Cramps
- Unusual Pain
- Ice Pick Pain
- Headache
- Light Sensitivity
- Red Eyes
- Blurred Vision
- Tearing
- Sinus Problems
- Cough
- Shortness of Breath
- Abdominal Pain
- Diarrhea
- Joint Pain
- Morning Stiffness
- Memory Issues
- Focus/Concentration Issues
- Word Recollection Issues
- Decreased Learning of New Knowledge
- Confusion
- Disorientation
- Skin Sensitivity
- Mood Swings
- Appetite Swings
- Sweats (especially night sweats)
- Temperature Regulation Problems
- Excessive Thirst
- Increased Urination
- Static Shocks
- Numbness
- Tingling
- Vertigo
- Metallic Taste
- Tremors

LYME DISEASE

Lyme disease is a vector-born disease contracted from the bite of a small tick, transmitting the spiral-shaped bacteria (spirochete) *Borrelia burgdorferi*. As the International Lyme and Associated Diseases Society (ILADS) states, "Ticks know no borders and respect no boundaries. A patient's county of residence does not accurately reflect his or her Lyme disease risk because people travel, pets travel, and ticks travel. This creates a dynamic situation with many opportunities for exposure to Lyme disease for each individual." There were two hundred thousand newly diagnosed cases of Lyme disease in 2017 alone, making it the fasting growing infectious disease in the United States (Smith 2017).

Not everyone with Lyme disease remembers their tick bite, or presents with the classic red bullseye rash (erythema migrans). In fact 30–40 percent of adults with confirmed Lyme never have a rash (Smith 2017). I have had patients come to me with classic textbook symptoms of Lyme, including the rash, joint pain, and headache. I have also had patients without the classic symptoms, who have instead had more vague symptoms, like brain fog and fatigue. Other symptoms reported by patients include flu-like symptoms, fever, aches, stiffness, jaw discomfort, swollen glands, red eyes, and even paralysis. Symptoms can appear, disappear, and then reappear (IGeneX 2017). Lyme disease has been called the "great mimicker." Many patients with diagnoses of chronic fatigue syndrome, fibromyalgia, somatization disorder, multiple sclerosis, and other difficult-to-diagnose multisystem illnesses could be experiencing a result of an undetected infection like Lyme. Diagnosis is based on symptoms, tick exposure, and labs.

The Centers for Disease Control (CDC) currently recommends a two-step process to test for evidence of antibodies against the Lyme disease bacteria. An enzyme-linked immunosorbent assay, also called **ELISA**, or **EIA**, is a test that can detect and measure antibodies in your blood. The first step in this testing process is to check the EIA, or rarely, an IFA (indirect immunofluorescence assay). If this first step is negative, no further testing of the specimen is recommended.

However, if the first step is positive or indeterminate (sometimes called "equivocal"), the second step should be performed. The second step uses a test called an immunoblot test, or, commonly, a Western blot test. Results are considered positive only if the EIA/IFA and the immunoblot are both positive.

According to the CDC, oral antibiotics commonly used for treatment include doxycycline, amoxicillin, or cefuroxime. The conventional treatment is a few weeks of the antibiotic doxycycline. However, I have not seen a study demonstrating that only fourteen to twenty-eight days of antibiotic treatment always cures Lyme disease. European medical studies show that short-term treatments have failed to eradicate the organism and that relapses of Lyme occur in 40 percent of cases, which can be devastating (ilads.org 2017).

Some providers believe many patients are either undertreated or misdiagnosed. The problem is availability of testing. Of all chronic infection labs, testing for Lyme is the most unreliable. The aforementioned EIA or ELISA test misses 35 percent of culture-proven Lyme cases, rendering it unacceptable for many providers. Many patients remain seronegative on Western blot testing. Also, antibodies to Lyme can decline over time, which can mean if a patient is not tested for Lyme until years past his exposure, they could test negative due to low antibodies in their blood.

The International Lyme and Associated Diseases Society (ILADS) is a nonprofit, international, multidisciplinary medical society dedicated to the appropriate diagnosis and treatment of Lyme and associated diseases. ILADS promotes understanding of these diseases through research, education, and policy. It strongly supports physicians, scientists, researchers and other health care professionals dedicated to advancing the standard of care for Lyme and associated diseases. To learn more, visit www.ilads.org.

According to the ILADS, a more accurate way to detect Lyme is to order a Western blot performed by a laboratory that reads and reports all of the bands related to *Borrelia burgdorferi* (ilads.org 2017). It's also important to test for other tick-transmitted coinfections, including *Babesia, Anaplasma, Ehrlichia,* and *Bartonella,* since "their continued presence increases morbidity and prevents successful treatment of Lyme disease" (ilads.org 2017).

Lyme disease can be devastating. If left untreated, this infection can spread to the joints, heart, and the nervous system. When that occurs, IV antibiotics are often required. Before I had patients with Lyme disease visit my clinic, I saw the documentary *Under Our Skin,* which was actually quite disturbing. I nearly became "lymeophobic," if such a term even exists. I saw how debilitating and life changing untreated Lyme can be. I was scared of Lyme, checking for ticks after every time I was outside (as we all should). My fear over the years has lessened, but my passion to help these patients has soared. Many of these patients also struggle with yeast overgrowth, due to the loads of antibiotics they have taken.

IGeneX is a very progressive lab started by Nick Harris, MD, who also helped form the ILADS society. The lab is a leader in developing tests to accurately detect Lyme disease, relapsing fever, and associated tick-borne diseases. IGeneX can test for Lyme disease several ways using two strains of *B. burgdorferi*. This allows detection of most *B. burgdorferi* infections (Lyme) in the United States, Canada, Europe, and Australia.

The lab can also test for various coinfections like babesiosis, bartonellosis, ehrlichiosis, and rickettsiosis. Many bands are not reported on the current basic Lyme test at your local lab. IGeneX tests for several additional bands.

There's no perfect test for Lyme diagnosis and treatment. It can be very complicated to diagnose and treat. When it is detected and treated, patients with Lyme disease also need to follow every step in the Longevity Blueprint simultaneously. To find a Lyme literate doctor near you, or to learn more about evidence-based treatment guidelines, visit the International Lyme and Associated Diseases Society website, www.ilads.org.

If patients have completed treatment of Lyme and have not improved, mold should be a seriously explored consideration.

MOLD

Contaminants found in the air and dust of water-damaged buildings can contribute to chronic inflammatory response syndrome (CIRS). Water intrusion in a home should be stopped and dried out within forty-eight hours. Not only can mold and bacteria grow on damp building materials, which is often visible, but it can also produce metabolites, which are not visible, and which can settle in the dust or become airborne. When you inhale these very small particles, the biotoxins enter your bloodstream and get delivered to your lungs, brain, muscles, and liver. One hundred thousand biotoxins can be found in a space as small as a period. If you can't clear these contaminants, they can wreak havoc on your body and trigger a huge cascade of inflammation (Berndtson 2016). In other words, biotoxins from water damaged buildings can be a source of CIRS, because WDBs contain a toxic stew of fungi, bacteria, mycobacteria, and actinomyces not just due to flooding. This is often due to construction defects like inappropriate heating, ventilation and air conditioning (HVAC) systems, faulty construction crawl spaces, or inadequate designs like having a flat roof, fake stucco cladding, inappropriate caulking, or poor water remediation.

Don't think you have been exposed to mold? The World Health Organization estimates that 50 percent of built environments in developed countries have suffered these damp conditions (Afshari et al. 2009). Did you grow up in an old, moldy home? Have you ever lived or worked in a water-damaged environment? I can list handfuls of individuals who didn't realize they had water damage in their home until they looked for it. What about your place of work? An office building analysis indicated that 30 to 50 percent of office environments in the United States have suffered water damage (Mendell 2005). How do you know if your home or office building carries these toxins? You test the environment—more on this to come.

What are other sources of these toxins? Food and drink. You must remove the exposure in your home and also in your foods. Grains like wheat and corn, fruits, chocolate, wine, and peanuts can all be contaminated with mold toxins. Obviously, dairy products such as cheese can contain mold, because the cows that produce the milk may have consumed contaminated grains.

One major source of these toxins that David Asprey, founder of Bulletproof Coffee, has studied is coffee. The amount of mold toxins can vary from batch to batch. Other countries have actually instituted rules for how much of these toxins is acceptable. The United States, however, has no such rules. Decaf has more mold toxins, because, as the caffeine is removed, the beans are left defenseless against mold (Asprey 2014).

Asprey also discusses other toxins, like ochratoxins (OTA), a class of several different chemicals belonging to the fungal toxins known as mycotoxins. In his book, *The Bulletproof Diet*, Asprey shares that *Aspergillus ochraceus*, in particular, contaminates dried foods, but more importantly seems to be the culprit, along with *Aspergillus niger*, for contaminating green coffee beans. In case you are wondering, roasting kills the mold, but the mold toxin—the OTA—remains. Asprey states that as much as 58 percent of coffee beans are contaminated, and that regular coffee consumption can contribute to mold toxicity. This can lead to heart failure, cancer, high blood pressure, kidney disease, and brain damage. Mold also makes you more food sensitive. Cleansing your body of mold may allow for more tolerance of other foods. Asprey has created a bulletproof coffee without ochrotoxins. To learn more, view his documentary *Moldy*, and to purchase his coffee visit www.bulletproof.com.

TESTING FOR CIRS

For patients with suspected biotoxin illnesses causing CIRS, the commonly ordered inflammatory tests, including a sedimentation rate (sed rate), antinuclear antibodies (ANA), C-reactive protein, lymphocytes, and CBC, can return normal. The patient can be told they are normal, even though they may clearly be suffering from multiple symptoms in multiple body systems. However, a well-trained provider can explore further testing. These patients often have high complement component 4A (C4a), high matrix (MMP-9), high transforming growth factor beta 1 (TGF beta-1), low melanocyte-stimulating hormone (MSH), low antidiuretic hormone (ADH), abnormal vascular endothelial growth factor (VEGF), and low vasoactive intestinal peptide (VIP). C4a responds to toxins made by living things. It aggressively initiates a cascade of downstream markers. Complement C3a (C3a) is an anaphylatoxin. It is elevated with Lyme disease and other tick borne illnesses. It is often low with mold cases. To complicate things, guess what all these abnormal labs lead to: low sex hormones (discussed in chapter 6).

Remember chapter 3, on genetics? Want to know if you are in that 25 percent of the population who can't clear biotoxins from Lyme and mold very well? Have your provider run the HLA DR/

DQ genotyping that shows if an individual has increased susceptibility to mold and Lyme.

Visual contrast sensitivity testing (VCS) is another way to assess differences in shading, thickness, and separation of hash marks. Over 90 percent of patients with CIRS will fail a VCS test, since they tend to have a weakness of the arterial supply in the upper outer portions of their optic nerves, where edge detection is located. You can take this test at www.survivingmold.com.

Shoemaker has an evidenced-based treatment protocol involving several steps, and has written more than six books on this topic already. I'm only covering the basics here. Treatment begins with the total removal of exposure to the contaminants, and remediation without delay. This may mean leaving your home and throwing away your books and clothes. The recommended testing per Shoemaker's protocol includes the Environmental Relative Moldiness Index (ERMI), as well as the Health Effects Roster of Type Specific Formers of Mycotoxins and Inflammagens, verse 2 (HERTSMI-2). If you'd like to test your home or office, testing options can be found at www.mycometrics.com/online.html. Learn more about how to collect this test at www.biotoxinhelp.com. Again, an experienced provider can help guide you through this.

CHRONIC VIRUSES

Not only can biotoxins cause major issues for patients, viruses can also be the source of many chronic illnesses, including fibromyalgia, chronic fatigue syndrome, and autoimmune disorders like multiple sclerosis, rheumatoid arthritis, Hashimoto's, and lupus.

The more patients I test, the more common I realize viruses are. Here are just a few of the more common ones.

Epstein-Barr Virus (EBV) is actually one of the herpetic viruses. It's commonly referred to as the mono virus, and is more common in run-down high-schoolers. This is the virus that makes you very tired, and can enlarge the spleen, which requires six weeks off from any sport activities. We are now finding that these viruses can become reactivated later in life. Additionally, heavy metals can be fuels for viruses, specifically arsenic, lead, and mercury. One theory is that since the thyroid can attract heavy metals, the virus can migrate there, causing Hashimoto's and eventually hypothyroidism.

Parvovirus infection is more prominent in children. It's often called the slapped-cheek disease, because of the distinctive face rash that develops on the cheeks. It's one of the five common childhood illnesses, which is why it has also been called fifth disease.

Cytomegalovirus (CMV) is common in adults and children. It can cause fever, sore throat, fatigue, and swollen glands. It can also cause mono or hepatitis.

Nearly everyone reading this has likely had several viruses in their lives, including the **varicella-zoster virus (VZV)**, also known as **chicken pox**. This is a contagious disease, causing blister-like rashes, itching, tiredness, and fever. The rash often starts on the stomach, spreads to the back and face, and can eventually spread to the entire body.

Usually occurring in older adults with weakened immune systems due to stress, injury, or medications, the VZV can reactivate, causing a very painful rash called **shingles**. This usually manifests in a stripe across one part of the body (along a dermatome).

Human Herpes Virus 6 (HHV6) has been associated with chronic fatigue syndrome. It has been found in the uterus of women with infertility and in the thyroid of individuals with Hashimoto's. It is also a suspected trigger for autoimmune diseases such as multiple sclerosis.

Hepatitis means inflammation of the liver. There are three well-known viral types: hepatitis A, B, and C. If left untreated, hepatitis can lead to liver cancer.

Human papillomavirus (HPV) was given its name for the papillomas, or warts, it can cause. Some types of HPV can lead to cancer of the mouth or throat, anus, rectum, penis, cervix, or vaginal and vulvar areas.

Viruses can be difficult to test for. Typically, ordered antibody panels can show past exposure, and medical providers oftentimes then interpret the results as past exposure only. More comprehensive testing can help deduce whether the virus has become reactivated. However, there are no tests to show where the viruses have become reactivated (Medical Medium 2017). *All* viruses can reactivate. Your goal is to keep your total viral count or load down, lessening the chance for recurrence.

I find my complex patients to have a bad combination of poor gut health, nutritional deficiencies, hormone imbalances, and poor genetic makeup, as well as a burden of various biotoxins and viruses. This is precisely why many chronic conditions are so very difficult to treat and resolve.

SUPPLEMENTS TO STRENGTHEN THE IMMUNE SYSTEM

Although this book doesn't focus on sleep or exercise, both are crucial to ensuring a strong immune system. As previously mentioned, the start of building your healthy foundation involves eating clean. To strengthen your immune system, you should first limit processed foods, sugar, artificial sweeteners, artificial colors, and hydrogenated oils. Limit foods that are pro-inflammatory, and that further stress your body. In addition to gut healing, the bone broth mentioned in chapter 1 is also excellent for immune support. You can also make an immunity broth with two cups organic chicken broth, four chopped shallots, two chopped carrots, five shiitake mushrooms, two cloves of garlic, and two ounces cooking greens like chard, kale, spinach, or mustard greens. Using spices and herbs like garlic, ginger, and turmeric are excellent ways to boost your meals. Herbs like Echinacea, goldenseal, and ginseng are also known to contain immune boosting properties.

IMMUNITY BROTH RECIPE

Two cups organic chicken broth
Four chopped shallots
Two chopped carrots
Five shiitake mushrooms
Two cloves of garlic
Two ounces cooking greens like chard, kale, spinach, or mustard greens.

Olive leaf extract is antiviral, antifungal, and antibacterial. It is a well-known agent to help enhance thymus function. Remember, the thymus helps train our T cells. Olive leaf also contains anti-inflammatory and antioxidant properties. LB's NK Complex is a specifically designed formula to support the body's immune response by boosting natural killer (NK) cell activity. It contains olive leaf, arabinogalactins, aloe vera, and zinc. One way AIDS affects the immune system is to lower the efficiency of NK cells. Enhancing NK cell activity promotes the normal process of eliminating unhealthy cells.

Astragalus is an adaptogenic herb. This means it helps to protect the body against various stresses, including physical, mental, and emotional stresses. It contains antioxidants, which protects cells against damage and destruction. It can also be used to protect and support the immune system, preventing colds and upper respiratory infections, lowering blood pressure, treating diabetes, and protecting the liver. It has been known to enhance NK cells and lymphocytes. Astragalus has antibacterial and anti-inflammatory properties. It also helps the growth and development of every lymphoid organ (UMMC 2017).

As mentioned in previous chapters, you don't want to be vitamin D deficient. **Vitamin D** is not only important for your bones, it is typically one of the first supplements I recommend to my patients to help modulate both the innate and adaptive immune responses. Vitamin D deficiency is associated with increased autoimmunity, as well as an increased susceptibility to infection (Aranow 2011).

I use a **silver hydrosol** product in my functional medicine practice often. This is an antiviral, antifungal, and antibacterial agent. My clinic carries the Argentyn 23 product, which is a professional grade of silver hydrosol available only through licensed health care practitioners. It contains the smallest particles ever seen in colloidal silver products, with the most unique charge attributes (98 percent positively charged). This product can't turn you blue or gray. It won't accumulate in your tissues. It's easily excreted by the body. The maker, Natural Immunogenics, doesn't use additives or stabilizers, nor does the product contain salts or proteins (often used to keep silver in suspension, but which create silver compounds). It is pure, meaning it contains only 99.999 percent pure silver suspended in pharmaceutical-grade purified water. I take one teaspoon each morning for general immune support, holding it under my tongue for one to two minutes, then swallowing. Getting that silver into my system helps me fight off any organisms I may come into contact with. Silver is excellent for flu season. It can be taken several times a day *if* you feel like you are developing symptoms of the flu, or even respiratory infections. Progressive clinics that treat Lyme and other biotoxin illnesses use this product intravenously (IV) to eradicate the organisms.

Lauricidin® is pure sn-1 monolaurin (glycerol monolaurate) derived from coconut oil. I use this commonly in my patients with yeast and chronic viruses, slowly increasing their dose. Lauricidin destroys viral envelopes, making the viruses easier for your body to eliminate.

Probiotics are discussed in chapter 1 and are essential for general immune support. They line your mucous membranes with good bacteria to help keep invaders out. They can also increase NK cell and macrophage activity. They have been known to increase IgA, IgM, and IgG secreting cells, enhancing the cellular immune response.

Mushrooms have long been used for immune support. They can affects both the innate and adaptive responses. The top two mushrooms I use are chaga and reishe. Their beta-glucans increase the immune system's T-cell levels. They can also help activate B cells. Medicinal mushrooms can help to kill bacteria, viruses, and yeast. They have also been shown to limit cancer cell growth and spread of tumors.

Lastly, rather than take antihistamines and anti-inflammatories for allergy-related symptoms, taking **quercetin** can help prevent the mast cell from exploding, thus preventing not only the allergenic cascade and its negative symptoms but also preventing the need for medications. LB's Seasonal Assist Product is excellent for allergy prevention. This is different than DAO, discussed in chapter 1, which is an enzyme needed to degrade or break down histamine.

MEDICATIONS

Many patients suffering with Lyme disease require long-term oral or IV antibiotics. Some patients with chronic viruses also require use of pharmaceutical antivirals. Few medications exist to truly treat CIRS. The main goal with CIRS is to reduce the load and to bind the toxins to help them be eliminated, thereby reducing inflammation.

Cholestyramine is a common next step. Cholestyramine (CSM) is an FDA-approved medication used to lower elevated levels of cholesterol. It has been used safely for over forty years by patients who have taken the medication for extended periods of time. It's a glue that binds toxins tightly so that they can't be reabsorbed, because it can't be absorbed. It has a long backbone with side chains, each with a nitrogen atom and positive charge. It often needs to be compounded, since the commercially available form is full of additives and artificial sweeteners. It can be taken up to four times daily. I this use in my mold cases. Other specialized compounded medications like Bactroban, EDTA, Gentamycin (BEG) spray, and vasoactive intestinal polypeptide (VIP) spray can be prescribed when needed. **BEG** spray is used to help bust through biofilm, allowing antibiotics to synergistically kill the organisms needed when patients have **multiple antibiotic resistant coagulase negative staphylococcus** (MARCoNS) infecting their nasal cavities (common in biotoxin cases). **VIP** spray is used to stop increased inflammation and restore immune regulation. Its use is the very last step in Shoemaker's protocol. To learn more, visit www.survivingmold.com.

CONCLUSION

Great efforts have been made since our local floods to rebuild, only to evacuate again in 2016 when our river flooded once more. Fortunately, that time our city was more prepared. We no doubt have hundreds, possibly thousands, suffering with CIRS, unaware of their condition and still looking for answers.

Most of these patients with chronic infections require every step in this Longevity Blueprint. Many have terrible gut health, numerous nutritional deficiencies, and very low hormone levels contributing to why they feel so terrible. If your basement floods, or your roof leaks, you must follow proper remediation strategies to assure it is safe to return to. If you are in the 25 percent of the population that is genetically susceptible to these toxins, you may also need to see a provider who can diagnose and treat you for CIRS.

Becky had CIRS. She needed to remove herself from her home to remove her exposure. She was started on cholestyramine to bind up the toxins that had been recirculated in her body. Becky is now proud and thankful to finally be free of vertigo, brain fog, and diarrhea. Her health has dramatically improved. Fortunately, she had not yet developed autoimmune diseases. Sadly, that isn't the case with other complicated cases I've seen. Some women have several autoimmune diseases by the time they arrive at our clinic. My goal with my patients when we get to this step in the Longevity Blueprint is to prevent the progression of autoimmune diseases, remove the inflammatory biotoxins, and strengthen the immune system. Just think of all the barriers the human body has been created with. Just as we want a strong roof on our house, we need a strong immune system to keep invaders out. That is the most challenging step, but one that is required for many people to regain their health.

Taking support daily like vitamin D and silver is a great first step to keep your immune system strong. However, I encourage you to find a knowledgeable provider to test for chronic viruses and for other biotoxin-related illnesses. If you or your loved ones have been exposed to biotoxins, from water damaged buildings or even from vector borne illnesses like Lyme disease, please see a CIRS or Lyme specialist—the sooner the better. Don't let your roof allow invaders in. Or, if they are already in, work to get them out. You can strengthen your immune system by following your Longevity Blueprint.

Longevity Blueprint Nutraceutical Products

Here are my favorite LB nutrients.

- NK Complex
- Seasonal Assist
- Probiotic Complex (20 billion CFUs)
- Advanced Probiotic (100 billion CFUs)
- Probiotic Ultra (225 billion CFUs)

Chapter 8 Resources

Biotoxin CIRS Help: www.biotoxinhelp.com

IGeneX Inc.: www.igenex.com

International Lyme and Associated Diseases Society: http://www.ilads.org/

Natural Immunogenics: http://natural-immunogenics.com
Surviving Mold: www.survivingmold.com

The Lauricidin Company: www.lauricidin.com

Mycometrics: www.mycometrics.com

Chapter 8 References

1. Afshari, A., et al. "WHO guidelines for indoor air quality: dampness and mould." World Health Organization (2009). http://www.euro.who.int/__data/assets/pdf_file/0017/43325/E92645.pdf.

2. Aranow, C. "Vitamin D and the Immune System." *Journal of Investigative Medicine* 6. no. 59. (2011): 881–886.

3. Asprey, D. *The Bulletproof Diet.* New York: Rodale Books, 2014.

4. University of Maryland Medical Center. "Astragalus." umm.edu. Accessed 2017, http://umm.edu/health/medical/altmed/herb/astragalus.

5. Berndtson, Keith. "How to Assess and Treat Mold Toxicity." Lecture at SHEICON Conference (2016).

6. Berndtson, Keith, Scott McMahon, Mary Ackerley, Sonia Rapaport, Sandeep Gupta, and Ritchie C. Shoemaker. *Medically sound investigation and remediation of water-damaged buildings in case of chronic inflammatory response syndrome.* Center for Research on Biotoxin Associated Illness. Pocomoke: Maryland, 2016.

7. Medical Medium. "Epstein Barr Virus Revealed." medicalmedium.com. Accessed 2017, http://www.medicalmedium.com/blog/epstein-barr-virus-revealed.

8. Mendell, M.J. "Indoor environments and occupants' health. What do we know?" *Implementing Health-Protective Features and Practices in Buildings: Workshop Proceedings*. Federal Facilities Council Technical Report, no. 148, (2005).

9. Shoemaker, Ritchie. "What is Mold Illness? Better yet, do people get sick after being exposed to water-damaged buildings?" SurvivingMold (2011). http://www.survivingmold.com/diagnosis.

10. Smith, Pamela. "Lyme Testing and Therapies." Lecture. Lab Interpretation Conference. American Academy of Anti-Aging Medicine (2017).

CHAPTER 9

GETTING STARTED: FIND A CONTRACTOR, OR PROVIDER, WHO CAN HELP WITH YOUR BUILDING PROCESS

How do you achieve health and promote longevity? By committing to your Longevity Blueprint. You now know how to build a healthy gastrointestinal foundation. You have been introduced to a blueprint you can follow to restore your gut health, maintain your spine, influence genetics, replete nutritional deficiencies, and optimize your hormones. You know how important it is to detoxify, to reduce your cardiovascular risk, and to strengthen your immune system. Committing to your Longevity Blueprint will take a significant commitment, but the results can dramatically alter the remainder of your life.

INVEST FINANCIALLY IN YOUR HEALTH

Health is like money, we never have a true idea of its value until we lose it.

—Josh Billings

CHAPTER # AND TITLE	
1	YOUR FOUNDATION: RESTORING GUT HEALTH
2	MAINTAINING YOUR FRAMEWORK: KEEPING YOUR SPINE IN LINE
3	ELECTRICAL WORK: INFLUENCING YOUR GENETICS
4	HAVING THE KEYS TO UNLOCK DOORWAYS: REPLETING NUTRITIONAL DEFICIENCIES
5	TACKLING THE LAUNDRY: DETOXIFYING THE BODY
6	MANAGING YOUR HEATING/COOLING: OPTIMIZING YOUR HORMONES
7	CLOG FREE PLUMBING: REDUCING CARDIOVASCULAR DISEASE
8	MAINTAINING ROOF INTEGRITY: STRENGTHENING THE IMMUNE SYSTEM
9	GETTING STARTED: FINDING A CONTRACTOR, OR PROVIDER WHO CAN HELP WITH YOUR BUILDING PROCESS

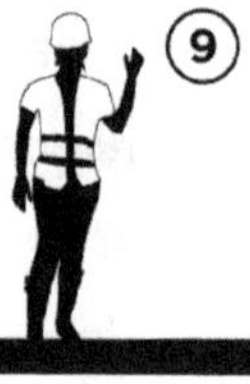

YOUR LONGEVITY BLUEPRINT

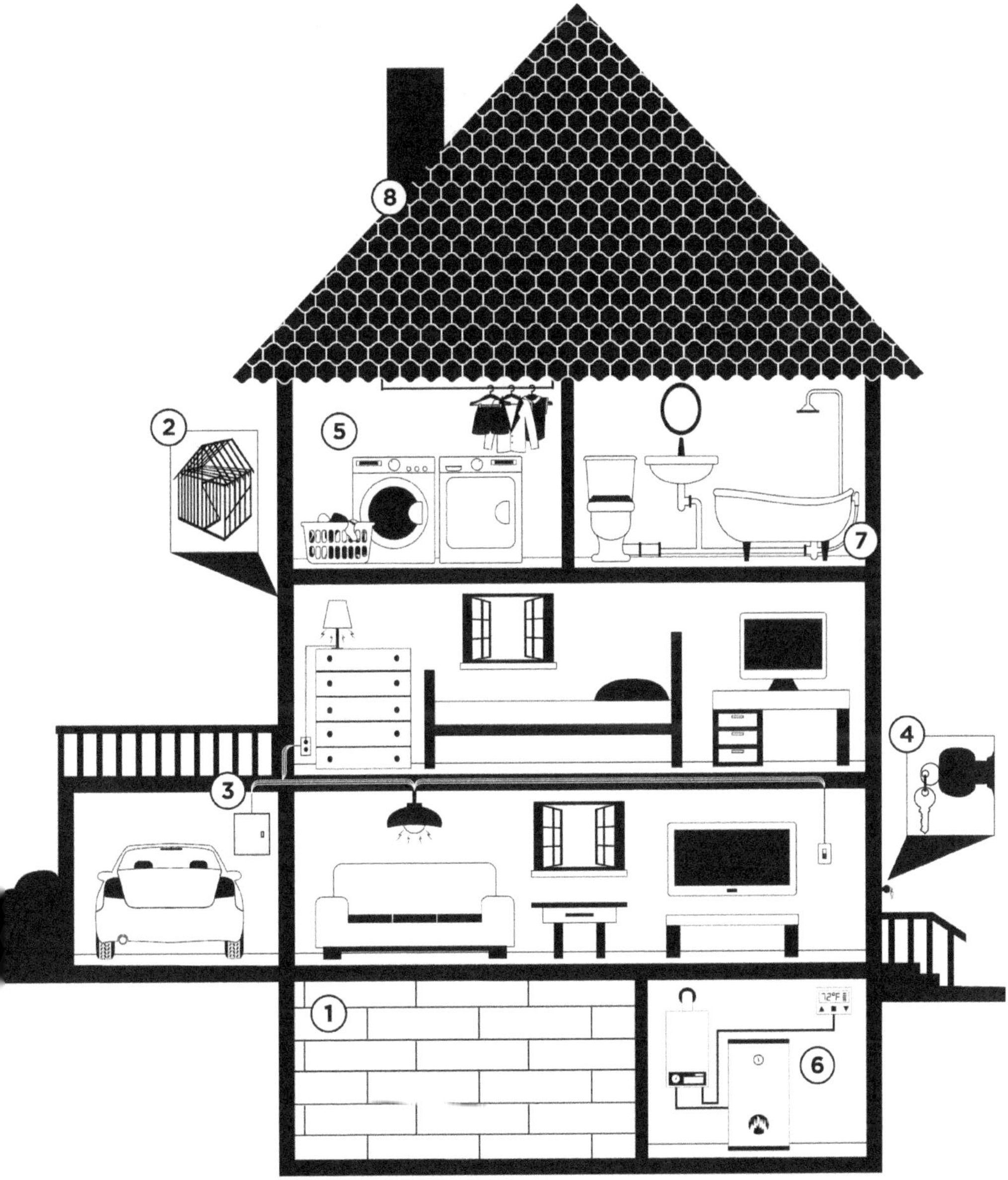
8
2
5
7
4
3
1
6

You need to invest financially in your health. Why, when diagnosed with cancer, is there no budget? People spend all their time, money, and resources to put out a fire, yet seldom put thought toward budgeting in prevention. Detecting breast cancer on a mammogram is not prevention. As mentioned earlier, the cost of CVD disease and stroke is $316 billion annually. The cost of diabetes is $245 billion annually and rising. Who is paying for this? We all are. We owe it to each other to take care of our bodies. That may mean spending money on a gym membership, on laboratory testing, and on vitamin D or probiotics, all items that your insurance will not cover.

FIND A CONTRACTOR

True health care reform starts in your kitchen, not in Washington.

—Anonymous

Part of your financial investment will be with your "contractor." I highly recommend you find a well-trained, experienced, functional medicine provider. Some of the most caring, inspiring, entrepreneurial individuals I know work within the integrative/functional/holistic sphere of medicine. Your contractor can help you work through the steps to longevity mentioned in this book to:

- restore gut health
- keep your spine in line
- influence your genetics
- replete nutritional deficiencies
- detoxify your body
- optimize your hormones

- reduce cardiovascular disease
- strengthen your immune system

LONGEVITY BLUEPRINT—SHIFTING THE PARADIGM

Most providers don't start out practicing functional medicine, working as a contractor. Most of these providers start practicing conventional medicine, putting out fires until one day conventional medicine is *unable* to help them, their family members, or their loved ones. At that point, their focus expands to what other approaches may be available. Many of these providers have their own personal stories, like I do. They may have struggled with their health, too, and now have refocused their lives on helping their patients use functional medicine.

A specialist is trained to focus on one system or organ within the body. We need these specialists within our health care systems, especially if surgical intervention is necessary. If you, as a patient, have a rare kidney condition, you absolutely need to see a nephrologist to put out that fire. If you need a brain tumor removed, you'd better go see a neurosurgeon, right? Sometimes surgery can be the most important intervention toward longevity. However, that specialist may not expand their focus to connecting the dots to what led to the health abnormality. Why? It's not always because the specialist doesn't want to know what caused the brain tumor. The expertise that is required to be a surgeon in any form is a profound skill set that takes years of training. Personally, I want my surgeon to have a laser-like focus on whatever it is they're operating on.

The issue is that surgery is not always necessary. If you need to have your fires put out, please get them put out, but if you want to get to the root cause of your health problems, find a functional medicine provider—someone who can be a detective to get to the root cause of your problem. Conventional medicine has specialists that focus on each system within the body. Functional medicine uses diagnostic testing that focuses on each system within the body. The test results act as the organ system specialists, and the results obtained from this testing provide the materials to **build true longevity**.

Visit the following websites to see if there is a provider in your area certified in anti-aging or functional medicine: www.A4M.com (antiaging, regenerative, and functional medicine), www.IFM.org (functional medicine), www.seekinghealth.org (genetics/MTHFR).

You can see how complex assessing for biotoxin illnesses can be. If you think you are suffering from a biotoxin illness, find a provider who specializes in that. Visit www.survivingmold.com (Lyme, mold, chronic inflammatory response syndrome) or visit the International Lyme and Associated Diseases Society's provider database at http://ilads.org/ilads_media/physician-referral/.

INVEST IN LIFESTYLE AND DIETARY CHANGES

A man too busy to take care of his health is like a mechanic too busy to take care of his tools.
—Spanish proverb

As part of your Longevity Blueprint, you will need to invest in lifestyle changes. There's no order of importance here. Eating clean, physical fitness, and managing stress are all equally important. You can never be too busy to take care of yourself. Are you loading up on caffeine all day and not drinking any water? How much alcohol are you stressing your liver with? How much toxic makeup and deodorant are you using?

You also need to invest in dietary changes. You may need to give up your favorite food—even if it's cheese. The best way to reduce inflammation is to remove those triggers that are often the foods we are eating.

You will need to complete the appropriate testing to help determine your triggers, to help determine what hormones you need balanced and the nutrients you need to take. This is exactly what I did and continue to do with my patients.

COMPLETE RECOMMENDED TESTING

As you can see, with all that I have mentioned in this book, there are several valuable testing options available to you. These tests are likely not going to be available through your primary care provider. Would you consult with a plumber to complete your electrical work? Certainly not. Similarly, you need to see a functional medicine specialist for this type of testing. You may think you are low in estrogen only to find out you're low in progesterone. Testing helps confirm what your risk factors may be. You can't always "feel" that you have a cardiovascular disease working to clog your arteries, or that you have an autoimmune disease. Testing leaves the guesswork out.

REGULARLY TAKE YOUR NECESSARY NUTRACEUTICAL PRODUCTS

Pending your nutritional testing results, you will need to commit to your recommended nutrient schedule. Remember, as mentioned in chapter 4, foods no longer provide all the nutrients required for optimal functioning. Living in Iowa (not the sunshine state) we are all more likely to have low vitamin D levels and omega-3 indexes, as we don't have access to fresh fish. Pending your genetic testing, you may be predisposed to poor detoxification and may need to take nutrients to help facilitate this.

CONCLUSION

The greatest wealth is health.
—Unknown

It will cost you, your family, your friends, and our health care system billions of dollars if we don't help to educate each other on what health truly is.

We all need this blueprint, so thank you for taking the time to read this book.

Remember, your family doctor can't walk you through the Longevity Blueprint. They don't have the education or training in this approach. They don't have access to all the labs. Most work for organizations that understandably want to profit off their labs and thus require that labs be run through their own organizations. They don't have contracts with all the specialty functional medicine labs providers like myself do. They don't have access to the necessary high-quality nutraceutical products.

Find a provider to help you. Remember, you need a contractor, a builder, who can assess what I've called your **fingerprint, your test results**, to help you get your body functioning the best it can. True health exists when all your organs are functioning to the best of their abilities. Imagine being excited to visit your doctor's office, to see your contractor, who can help you get to the root cause of your problems, a provider authentically interested in helping you, not only relying on drugs and surgery. As my chiropractor and friend Calla Jayne Kleene would say, "Let's make healthy contagious!" Tying health into longevity, I say, "Let's make Longevity contagious!"

Let's make Longevity contagious!

I hope this book has empowered you to make informed choices with the provider you seek, and to invest in the recommended testing. I hope it will inspire you to change your eating and take the nutrients you need. Isn't that the best advice for longevity—assessing and personalizing your care?

I'm no longer struggling with tachycardia. I have been able to identify my triggers with knowledge of my genetics. I take Magnesium Chelate and Mitochondrial Complex daily, and use L theanine when stressed. I'm on a high salt, gluten-free, lower FODMAP diet; I take all my necessary nutrients daily; I detox twice annually; I have optimized my hormones; I have resolved my SIBO. I will always continue to see my chiropractor. I will continuously work to reduce my stress and strengthen my immune system. As you can see, following the Longevity Blueprint gave me my life back. It was the best investment I've ever made, and can be yours, too.

Visit my practice website where you can view testimonials of individuals who have worked through our blueprint at www.ihhclinic.com, and visit www.yourlongevityblueprint.com for the LB products discussed throughout the book. You will also find free resources to accompany this book.

We are so very thankful for our patients and followers who have made this Longevity Blueprint possible. Please share this book with your family and friends.

Let's live long together! What are you waiting for?

WELLNESS IS WAITING™!

INDEX

B

C

D

G

H

X

Y

Z

CPSIA information can be obtained
at www.ICGtesting.com
Printed in the USA
BVHW080923251119
564754BV00023B/1271/P

9 781599 328591